NORTHERN DEVON HEALTHCARE
Library - Barnstaple

Advanced Cardiac Life Support

Advanced Cardiac Life Support
A Guide for Nurses

Second Edition

Phil Jevon

RGN, BSc (Hon), PGCE, ENB 124
Resuscitation Officer/Clinical Skills Lead
Honorary Clinical Lecturer
Manor Hospital
Walsall
UK

Consulting Editor
Dr Jagtar Singh Pooni
BSc (Hon), FRCA, FRCP
Consultant in Anaesthesia and Intensive Care Medicine
New Cross Hospital
Wolverhampton
UK

 WILEY-BLACKWELL

A John Wiley & Sons, Ltd., Publication

This edition first published 2010
© 2002, 2010 Phil Jevon

Blackwell Publishing was acquired by John Wiley & Sons in February 2007. Blackwell's publishing programme has been merged with Wiley's global Scientific, Technical, and Medical business to form Wiley-Blackwell.

First published 2002 by Butterworth-Heinemann
Second edition published 2010 by Wiley-Blackwell

Registered office
John Wiley & Sons Ltd, The Atrium, Southern Gate, Chichester, West Sussex, PO19 8SQ, United Kingdom

Editorial offices
9600 Garsington Road, Oxford OX4 2DQ, United Kingdom
2121 State Avenue, Ames, Iowa 50014-8300, USA

For details of our global editorial offices, for customer services and for information about how to apply for permission to reuse the copyright material in this book please see our website at www.wiley.com/wiley-blackwell.

The right of the author to be identified as the author of this work has been asserted in accordance with the Copyright, Designs and Patents Act 1988.

Wiley also publishes its books in a variety of electronic formats. Some content that appears in print may not be available in electronic books.

Designations used by companies to distinguish their products are often claimed as trademarks. All brand names and product names used in this book are trade names, service marks, trademarks or registered trademarks of their respective owners. The publisher is not associated with any product or vendor mentioned in this book. This publication is designed to provide accurate and authoritative information in regard to the subject matter covered. It is sold on the understanding that the publisher is not engaged in rendering professional services. If professional advice or other expert assistance is required, the services of a competent professional should be sought.

Library of Congress Cataloging-in-Publication Data
Jevon, Philip.
    Advanced cardiac life support : a guide for nurses / Phil Jevon.
        p. ; cm.
    Includes bibliographical references and index.
    ISBN 978-1-4051-8566-0 (pbk. : alk. paper)   1. Cardiovascular system–Diseases–Nursing.   2. Cardiac intensive care.   I. Title.
    [DNLM: 1. Advanced Cardiac Life Support–methods.   2. Advanced Cardiac Life Support–nursing.   3. Nursing Care–methods.   WG 205 J58a 2010]
    RC674.J48 2010
    616.1'0231–dc22

                                                            2009013262

A catalogue record for this book is available from the British Library.

Set in 10/12 pt Palatino by SNP Best-set Typesetter Ltd., Hong Kong
Printed and bound in Malaysia by KHL Printing Co Sdn Bhd

1   2010

Contents

Acknowledgements

I am grateful to the following:

Dr Jagtar Singh Pooni, Consultant Anaesthetist and Intensivist, The Royal Wolverhampton NHS Trust, for kindly agreeing to be the consulting editor for the book.

Dr Shameer Gopal, Consultant Anaesthetist and Intensivist, The Royal Wolverhampton NHS Trust, for his help with the therapeutic hypothermia guidelines in Chapter 13.

Dr Jagtar Singh Pooni for updating Chapter 6, Airway Management and Ventilation, and Chapter 13, Post-Resuscitation Care.

Rebecca McBride, Senior Sister CCU, Manor Hospital, Walsall, for writing Chapter 11, Acute Coronary Syndromes.

Elaine Walton, Resuscitation Officer, Manor Hospital Walsall, for updating Chapter 15, Ethical Issues in Resuscitation.

Shareen Juwle and Steve Webb for their help with the photographs.

Magenta Lampson and her colleagues at Wiley-Blackwell for their help with the production and publication process.

Chapter 1

Resuscitation Service: An Overview

Introduction

Every hospital has a duty of care to ensure that an effective and safe resuscitation service is provided for its patients. The satisfactory performance of the resuscitation service has wide-ranging implications in terms of resuscitation equipment, resuscitation training, standards of care, clinical governance, risk management and clinical audit (Jevon, 2002; Royal College of Anaesthetists *et al.*, 2008). Standards for resuscitation and resuscitation training have been published (Royal College of Anaesthetists *et al.*, 2008).

The aim of this chapter is to provide an overview to the resuscitation service in the hospital setting.

Learning outcomes

At the end of the chapter the reader will be able to:

- Discuss the concept of the chain of survival
- Summarise *Cardiopulmonary Resuscitation: Standards for Clinical Practice and Training*
- Discuss the key recommendations in the joint statement
- Discuss the principles of safer handling during cardiopulmonary resuscitation (CPR)

Concept of the chain of survival

Survival from cardiac arrest relies on a sequence of time-sensitive interventions (Nolan *et al.*, 2006). The concept of the original chain of survival emphasises that each time-sensitive intervention

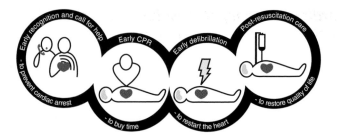

Fig. 1.1 Chain of survival. Reproduced with permission from Laerdal Medical Ltd, Orpington, Kent, UK.

must be optimised in order to maximise the chance of survival: a chain is only as strong as its weakest link (Cummins *et al.*, 1991).

The chain of survival was revised in 2005 (Figure 1.1) to stress the importance of recognising critical illness and/or angina and preventing cardiac arrest (both in and out of hospital) and post-resuscitation care (Nolan, 2005):

- *Early recognition and call for help to prevent cardiac arrest*: this link stresses the importance of recognising patients at risk of cardiac arrest, calling for help and providing effective treatment to hopefully prevent cardiac arrest; up to 80% of patients sustaining an in-hospital cardiac arrest have displayed signs of deterioration prior to collapse (Nolan *et al.*, 2006); most patients sustaining an out-of-hospital cardiac arrest also display warning symptoms for a significant duration before the event (Muller *et al.*, 2006)
- *Early CPR to buy time and early defibrillation to restart the heart*: the two central links in the chain stress the importance of linking CPR and defibrillation as essential components of early resuscitation in an attempt to restore life
- *Post-resuscitation care to restore quality of life*: the priority is to preserve cerebral and myocardial function, to restore quality of life and indicates the potential benefit that may be provided by therapeutic hypothermia

(Nolan *et al.*, 2006)

Cardiopulmonary Resuscitation: Standards for Clinical Practice and Training

Cardiopulmonary Resuscitation: Standards for Clinical Practice and Training (Royal College of Anaesthetists *et al.*, 2008) is a joint statement from the Royal College of Anaesthetists, Royal College of Physicians of London, Intensive Care Society and Resuscitation Council (UK). It has been endorsed by a number of national bodies, including the Royal College of Nursing and builds on previous reports and guidelines including those from the Royal College of Physicians and Resuscitation Council (UK) (Royal College of Anaesthetists *et al.*, 2008).

The joint statement makes a number of recommendations relating to:

- The resuscitation committee
- The resuscitation officer
- Resuscitation training
- Prevention of cardiopulmonary arrest
- The resuscitation team
- Resuscitation in children, pregnancy and trauma
- Resuscitation equipment
- Decisions relating to CPR
- Patient transfer and post-resuscitation care
- Audit and reporting standards
- Research

Key recommendations in the joint statement

Resuscitation committee
Each hospital should have a resuscitation committee that meets on a regular basis and is responsible for implementing operational policies relating to resuscitation practice and training. The chairperson should be a senior clinician who is actively involved in resuscitation. Membership of the committee should include:

- A physician
- A senior resuscitation officer
- An anaesthetist/intensivist
- A senior manager

- Representatives from appropriate departments, for example, accident and emergency (A&E), paediatrics, based on local needs

Responsibilities of the resuscitation committee include:

- Advising on the composition and role of the resuscitation team
- Ensuring that resuscitation equipment and resuscitation drugs are available
- Ensuring the adequate provision of resuscitation training
- Ensuring that Resuscitation Council (UK) guidelines and standards for resuscitation are followed
- Updating resuscitation and anaphylaxis policies
- Recording and reporting clinical incidents related to resuscitation
- Auditing resuscitation attempts and do not attempt resuscitation (DNAR) orders

Resuscitation officer

Each hospital should have a resuscitation officer responsible for resuscitation training, ideally one for every 750 clinical staff. The resuscitation officer should possess a current Resuscitation Council (UK) advanced life support (ALS) certificate and should ideally be a Resuscitation Council (UK) ALS instructor. Adequate training facilities, training equipment and secretarial support should be provided. Responsibilities of the resuscitation officer include:

- Implementing Resuscitation Council (UK) guidelines and standards in resuscitation
- Providing adequate resuscitation training for relevant hospital personnel
- Ensuring there are systems in place for checking and maintaining resuscitation equipment
- Auditing resuscitation attempts using the current Utstein template
- Attending resuscitation attempts and providing feedback to team members
- Coordinating participation in resuscitation-related trials
- Keeping abreast of current resuscitation guidelines

Resuscitation training

Clinical staff should receive regular (at least annual) resuscitation training appropriate to their level and expected clinical responsibilities. It should also be incorporated in the induction programme for new staff. The training should include the recognition and effective treatment of critical illness and providing effective treatment to prevent cardiopulmonary arrest. Some staff, e.g. members of the cardiac arrest team, will require appropriate advanced resuscitation training, e.g. Resuscitation Council (UK) Advanced Life Support (ALS) Course (see Chapter 17).

Extended nursing roles in resuscitation should be encouraged – for example, airway adjuncts, intravenous cannulation and administration of specific emergency drugs, electrocardiogram (ECG) interpretation and defibrillation.

The resuscitation officer is responsible for organising and coordinating the training; a cascade system of training may be needed to meet training demands, particularly in basic life support. Help should be sought from other medical and nursing specialities to provide specific training, such as in neonatal resuscitation.

See Chapter 17 for more detailed information on resuscitation training.

Prevention of cardiopulmonary arrest

Systems should be in place to identify patients who are critically ill and therefore at risk of cardiopulmonary arrest (Royal College of Anaesthetists *et al.*, 2008). Every hospital should have an early warning scoring system in place to identify these patients; adverse clinical indicators or scores should elicit a response to alert expert help, e.g. critical care outreach service, medical emergency team (National Institute for Health and Clinical Excellence (NICE), 2007).

Each healthcare organisation should have a patient's observation chart that facilitates the regular measurement and recording of early warning scores; there should be a clear and specific policy that requires a clinical response to 'calling criteria' or early warning systems ('track and trigger'), including the specific responsibilities of senior medical and nursing staff (Royal College of Anaesthetists *et al.*, 2008). For further information see Chapter 3.

The resuscitation team

Every hospital should have a resuscitation team. Ideally, this should include a minimum of two doctors who are trained in advanced life support. The resuscitation committee should advise on the composition of the cardiac arrest team, but overall the team should be able to perform:

- Airway management (including tracheal intubation)
- Intravenous cannulation (including central venous access)
- Defibrillation (advisory and manual) and electrical cardioversion
- Drug administration
- Advanced techniques, e.g. external cardiac pacing and pericardiocentesis
- Appropriate skills for effective post-resuscitation care

The resuscitation team should have a team leader (usually a doctor), whose responsibilities include:

- Directing and coordinating the resuscitation attempt
- Ensuring the safety of the patient and the team
- Terminating the resuscitation attempt when indicated
- Communicating with the patient's relatives and other healthcare professionals
- Documenting the resuscitation attempt (including audit forms)

The resuscitation team should be alerted within 30 seconds of dialing 2222 (recommended telephone number for contacting switchboard following an in-hospital cardiac arrest) (National Safety Patient Agency (NSPA), 2004). The system should be tested on a daily basis.

Resuscitation in children, pregnancy and trauma

Children: ideally, there should be a separate paediatric resuscitation team, with the team leader having expertise and training in paediatric resuscitation. All staff who are involved with paediatric resuscitation should be encouraged to attend national paediatric courses, e.g. European Paediatric Advanced Life Support (PALS), Advanced Paediatric Life Support (APLS) and Newborn Life Support (NLS).

Pregnancy: an obstetrician and a neonatologist should be involved at an early stage; minimising vascular compression by the gravid uterus and early advanced airway intervention are paramount, together with early consideration for peri-mortem Caesarean section (see Chapter 9).

Trauma: hospitals that admit patients with major injuries should have a multi-disciplinary trauma team; in particular, advanced airway management skills may be required.

Resuscitation equipment

The resuscitation committee is responsible for advising on resuscitation equipment, which will largely depend on local requirements and facilities. Ideally, it should be standardised throughout the hospital. Resuscitation equipment is discussed in detail in Chapter 2.

Decisions relating to cardiopulmonary resuscitation

Every hospital should have a 'Do not attempt resuscitation' policy, which should be based on national guidelines (British Medical Association *et al.*, 2007). For further information see Chapter 15.

Patient transfer and post-resuscitation care

Complete recovery from a cardiac arrest is rarely immediate, and the return of spontaneous circulation is just the start, not the end, of the resuscitation attempt; the immediate post-resuscitation period is characterised by high dependency and clinical instability (Jevon, 2002). The patient will probably need to be transferred to a coronary care unit or critical care unit.

Prior to transfer, the patient should be stabilised as far as possible, although this should not delay definitive treatment. Where appropriate, relevant equipment, drugs and monitoring devices should be available. Relatives will need to be informed of the transfer. Policies should be in place relating to transfers within and between hospitals (Jevon, 2002). Patient transfer and post-resuscitation care are discussed in detail in Chapter 13.

Audit and reporting standards

To help ensure a high quality resuscitation service, each hospital should audit:

- Resuscitation attempt (using the Utstein template), including outcomes
- The availability and use of resuscitation equipment
- The availability of emergency drugs
- Do not attempt resuscitation orders
- Critical incidents which cause, or occur during, cardiopulmonary arrests
- Health and safety issues, including cleaning and decontamination of resuscitation training mannequins (following each training session)

Hospital management should be informed of any problems that arise; the local clinical governance lead should support the resuscitation committee to rectify any deficiencies in the service.

Research
Heathcare practitioners interested in undertaking resuscitation-related research, should be encouraged to do so. They should be advised to seek the advice and support of the local research ethics committee.

Role of the Resuscitation Council (UK)

The Resuscitation Council (UK) was formed in August 1981 by a group of medical practitioners from a variety of specialities who shared an interest in, and concern for, the subject of resuscitation.

Objectives

The aim of the Resuscitation Council (UK) is to facilitate education of both lay and healthcare professionals in the most effective methods of resuscitation appropriate to their needs by:

- Encouraging research into methods of resuscitation
- Studying resuscitation teaching techniques
- Establishing appropriate guidelines for resuscitation procedures
- Promoting the teaching of resuscitation as established in the guidelines

- Establishing and maintaining standards for resuscitation
- Fostering good working relations between all organisations involved in resuscitation and producing and publishing training aids and other literature concerned with the organisation of resuscitation and its teaching

Courses

In order to teach theoretical and practical resuscitation skills to healthcare professionals, the Resuscitation Council (UK) has developed a variety of advanced courses. Including advanced life support courses in adult, paediatric and newborn resuscitation, which are run at centres throughout the UK.

Further details and information on all the Resuscitation Council (UK) courses are available on its website, www.resus.org.uk.

Guidelines

The Resuscitation Council (UK) has established working parties to review protocols for basic, advanced, paediatric and newborn resuscitation. These are available in the guidelines section on www.resus.org.uk.

Research

The Resuscitation Council (UK)'s Research Committee has available funding to assist new resuscitation initiatives. For further information access www.resus.org.uk.

Project teams

The Resuscitation Council (UK) project teams are set up as required to produce new guidelines and reports on relevant resuscitation topics and these are published periodically by the Council (see http://www.resus.org.uk/SiteIndx.htm).

Principles of safer handling during CPR

Approximately 80% of cardiac arrests in hospital are neither sudden nor unpredictable. In these situations the possible need to undertake CPR should therefore before be identified and a risk assessment, in relation to handling, carried out following local protocols.

The Resuscitation Council (UK), in their publication *Guidance for Safer Handling during Resuscitation in Hospitals* (Resuscitation Council (UK), 2001), has issued guidelines concerning safer handling during CPR. A brief overview of these guidelines will now be provided.

Cardiac arrest on the floor

- If the patient has collapsed on the floor, perform CPR on the floor. If the area has restricted access, consider sliding the patient across the floor using sliding sheets. Use mobile screens if required
- Ventilation: kneel behind the patient's head ensuring the knees are shoulder-width apart, rest back to sit on the heels and lean forwards from the hips towards the patient's face
- Tracheal intubation: kneel behind the patient's head ensuring the knees are shoulder-width apart, rest back to sit on the heels and lean forwards from the hips over the patient's face. Resting the elbows on the floor may provide the practitioner with greater stability
- Chest compressions: kneel at the side of the patient, level with his chest and adopt a high kneeling position with the knees shoulder-width apart; position the shoulders directly over the patient's sternum and, keeping the arms straight, compress the chest ensuring the force for compressions results from flexing the hips
- Following CPR: transfer the patient from the floor using a hoist (preferable); if a hoist is unavailable or impractical, a manual lift will need to be considered (this is a high-risk procedure and should only be considered as a last resort)

Cardiac arrest on a bed, trolley or couch

- Remove any environmental hazards, ensure the bed brakes are on and lower cotsides if they are up
- Moving the patient into a supine position: if a sliding sheet is already under the patient use that; if not quickly insert one, if

possible, under the patient's hips/buttocks by rolling him on to his side and then slide him down the bed
- Ventilation and intubation: move the bed away from the wall and remove the backrest to allow access; stand at the top of the bed facing the patient with the feet in a walk/stand position and avoid prolonged static postures
- Chest compressions: ensure the bed is at a height which places the patient between the knee and mid-thigh of the practitioner performing chest compressions; stand at the side of the bed with the feet shoulder-width apart, position the shoulders directly over the patient's sternum and, keeping the arms straight, compress the chest ensuring the force for compressions results from flexing the hips; chest compressions can also be performed by kneeling with both knees on the bed
- CPR on a fixed-height bed, couch or trolley: if necessary stand on steps or a firm stool, with a non-slip surface and wide enough to permit the practitioner's feet to be shoulder-width apart; do not kneel on a couch or trolley

Cardiac arrest in a chair

- Lowering the patient to the floor: with two colleagues, preferably using a slide sheet, slide the patient on to the floor; one should be supporting the patient's head during the procedure

Cardiac arrest in the toilet

- Ensure the toilet door is kept open and access maintained
- Lowering the patient to the floor: with two colleagues, slide the patient on to the floor; one should be supporting the patient's head during the procedure

Cardiac arrest in the bath

- Perform risk assessment following local protocols
- *Pull the plug out*
- Ensure the bath floor is quickly dried prior to evacuation
- Follow local evacuation procedure

Chapter summary

Hospitals must provide an effective resuscitation service and must ensure all appropriate staff are adequately trained and regularly updated to a level compatible with their expected degree of competence (Jevon, 2002). Adhering to the standards in *Cardiopulmonary Resuscitation: Standards for Clinical Practice and Training* (Royal College of Anaesthetists *et al.*, 2008), which have been highlighted in this chapter, will help ensure a high-quality and safe resuscitation service.

References

British Medical Association, Resuscitation Council (UK), Royal College of Nursing (2007) *Decisions relating to cardiopulmonary resuscitation. A joint statement from the British Medical Association, the Resuscitation Council (UK) and the Royal College of Nursing*. BMA, London: updated November 2007.

Cummins R, Ornato J, Thies W, Pepe P (1991) Improving survival from sudden cardiac arrest: the 'chain of survival' concept. A statement for health professionals from the Advanced Cardiac Life Support Subcommittee and the Emergency Cardiac Care Committee, American Heart Association. *Circulation* **83**:1832–47.

Jevon P (2002) *Advanced Cardiac Life Support: a Practical Guide*. Butterworth Heinemann, Oxford.

Muller D, Agrawal R, Arntz H (2006) How sudden is sudden cardiac death? *Circulation* **114**:1146–50.

National Safety Patient Agency (NSPA) (2004) *Crash call* http://www.npsa.nhs.uk/patientsafety/alerts-and-directives/alerts/crash-call/ Accessed 14 July 2008.

National Institute for Health and Clinical Excellence (NICE) (2007) *Acutely Ill Patients In Hospital: Recognition of and Response to Acute Illness in Adults in Hospital*. NICE, London.

Nolan J (2005) European Resuscitation Council Guidelines for Resuscitation 2005. Section 1: Introduction. *Resuscitation* **67**(Suppl. 1): S3–6.

Nolan J, Soar J, Eikeland H (2006) Image in resuscitation: the chain of survival. *Resuscitation* **71**:270–1.

Royal College of Anaesthetists, Royal College of Physicians of London, Intensive Care Society, Resuscitation Council (UK) (2008) *Cardiopulmonary Resuscitation: Standards for Clinical Practice and Training. A Joint Statement from The Royal College of Anaesthetists, The Royal College of Physicians of London, The Intensive Care Society, The Resuscitation Council (UK)*. The Royal College of Anaesthetists, London.

Chapter 2

Resuscitation Equipment

Introduction

A speedy response is essential in the event of a cardiac arrest. Procedures should be in place to ensure that all the essential resuscitation equipment is immediately available, accessible and in good working order. A carefully set out and fully stocked cardiac arrest trolley is paramount.

The local resuscitation committee should advise on what resuscitation equipment should be available, taking into account anticipated workload, availability of resuscitation equipment in nearby departments and specialised local requirements (Resuscitation Council (UK), 2008). A list of recommended resuscitation equipment for use in adults is available the Resuscitation Council (UK) website: http://www.resus.org.uk/pages/eqipIHAR.htm.

The aim of this chapter is to discuss the provision of resuscitation equipment.

Learning outcomes

At the end of this chapter the reader will be able to:

- List the recommended minimum equipment for the management of an adult cardiac arrest
- Discuss the routine checking of resuscitation equipment
- Discuss the checking of resuscitation equipment following use

Recommended minimum equipment for the management of an adult cardiac arrest

The Resuscitation Council (UK) (2004) recommends the following minimum equipment for the management of an adult cardiac arrest.

Airway equipment

- Pocket mask with oxygen port (should be widely available in all clinical areas)
- Self-inflating resuscitation bag with oxygen reservoir and tubing (ideally, the resuscitation bag should be single use – if not, it should be equipped with a suitable filter)
- Clear face masks, sizes 3, 4 and 5
- Oropharyngeal airways, sizes 2, 3 and 4
- Nasopharyngeal airways, sizes 6 and 7
- Portable suction equipment
- Yankauer suckers
- Tracheal suction catheters, sizes 12 and 14
- Laryngeal mask airways (LMAs) (sizes 4 and 5), or ProSeal LMAs (sizes 4 and 5), or Combitube (small)
- Magill forceps
- Tracheal tubes – oral, cuffed, sizes 6, 7 and 8
- Gum elastic bougie or equivalent device
- Lubricating jelly
- Laryngoscope handles (×2) and blades (standard and long blade)
- Spare batteries for laryngoscope and spare bulbs (if applicable)
- Fixation for tracheal tube (e.g. ribbon gauze/tape)
- Scissors
- Selection of syringes
- Oxygen mask with reservoir (non-rebreathing) bag
- Oxygen cylinder
- Cylinder key

Circulation equipment

- Defibrillator (shock advisory module and or external pacing facility to be decided by local policy)

- Electrocardiogram (ECG) electrodes
- Defibrillation gel pads or self-adhesive defibrillator pads (preferred)
- Selection of intravenous cannulae
- Selection of syringes and needles
- Cannula fixing dressings and tapes
- Seldinger central venous catheter kit
- Intravenous infusion sets
- 0.9% sodium chloride – 1000 ml × 2
- Arterial blood gas syringes
- Tourniquet

Drugs

Immediately available prefilled syringes
- Adrenaline 1 mg (1:10 000) × 4
- Atropine 3 mg × 1
- Amiodarone 300 mg × 1

Other readily available drugs
- Intravenous injections:
  - Adenosine 6 mg × 10
  - Adrenaline 1 mg (1:10 000) × 4
  - Adrenaline 1 mg (1:1,000) × 2
  - Amiodarone 300 mg × 1
  - Calcium chloride 10 ml of 100 mg per ml × 1
  - Chlorphenamine 10 mg × 2
  - Furosemide 50 mg × 2
  - Glucose 10% 500 ml × 1
  - Hydrocortisone 100 mg × 2
  - Lignocaine 100 mg × 1
  - Magnesium sulphate 50% solution 2 g (4 ml) × 1
  - Midazolam 10 mg × 1
  - Naloxone 400 µg × 5
  - Normal saline 10 ml ampoules
  - Potassium chloride for injection
  - Sodium bicarbonate 8.4% solution 50 ml × 1
- Other medications/equipment:
  - Salbutamol (5 mg × 2) and ipratropium bromide (500 µg × 2) nebules
  - Nebuliser device and mask

　○ Glyceryl trinitrate spray
　○ Aspirin 300 mg

Additional items

- Clock
- Gloves/goggles/aprons
- Audit forms
- Sharps container and clinical waste bag
- Large scissors
- Alcohol wipes
- Blood sample bottles
- A sliding sheet or similar device should be available for safer handling

The resuscitation equipment should be stored on a standard cardiac arrest trolley (Figure 2.1). It should be spacious, sturdy,

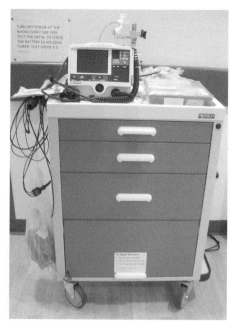

Fig. 2.1 A standard cardiac arrest trolley.

easily accessible and mobile. The layout of every cardiac arrest trolley in a hospital should ideally be standardised (Resuscitation Council (UK), 2009); this will help to minimise confusion. A defibrillator should also be immediately available. Where appropriate, e.g. general wards, it should have an automatic or advisory facility. Defibrillators with external pacing should be strategically located, e.g. accident and emergency (A&E), intensive therapy unit (ITU), coronary care unit (CCU).

Although piped or wall oxygen and suction should always be used when available, portable suction devices and oxygen should still be at hand either on or adjacent to the cardiac arrest trolley. Other items that the cardiac arrest team should have immediate access include a stethoscope, ECG machine, blood pressure measuring device, pulse oximeter, blood gas syringes and a device for verifying correct tracheal tube placement, e.g. oesophageal detector device (Resuscitation Council (UK), 2009).

Routine checking of resuscitation equipment

Resuscitation equipment should be routinely checked, ideally on a daily basis, by each ward or department with responsibility for the resuscitation trolley (Resuscitation Council (UK), 2009).

A system for daily documented checks of the equipment inventory should be in place. Some cardiac arrest trolleys can be 'sealed' with a numbered seal after being checked. Once the contents have been checked, the trolley can then be sealed and the seal number documented by the person who has checked the trolley. The advantage of this system is that an unbroken seal, together with the same seal number last recorded, signifies the trolley has not been opened since it was last checked and sealed. The equipment inventory should therefore be complete. A broken seal or an unrecorded seal number suggests the inventory may not be complete, hence a complete check is then required. The seal can easily be broken if the trolley needs to be opened.

Expiry dates should be checked, e.g. drugs, fluids, ECG electrodes, defibrillation pads. Laryngoscopes, including batteries and bulbs, should also be checked to ensure good working order. The self-inflating bag should be checked to ensure that there are no leaks and that the rim of the face mask is adequately inflated.

The defibrillator should be checked following the manufacturer's recommendations. This may involve charging up and discharging a shock into the defibrillator. Some defibrillators, e.g. automatic external defibrillators, perform self-checks on a daily basis. In addition, some defibrillators will need to remain plugged into the mains to ensure that the battery is fully charged in the event of use. It is recommended that advice is sought from a member of the Electro Biomedical Engineers (EBME) department or from the manufacturer's representative regarding how to undertake this.

Manufacturers usually recommend that ECG electrodes should be stored in their original packaging until immediately prior to use. However the policy at some hospitals is to leave them attached to the defibrillator leads. They should therefore be checked to ensure that the gel is moist, not dry. If they are dry they should be replaced.

All mechanical equipment, e.g. defibrillator, suction machine, should be inspected and serviced on a regular basis by the EBME department following the manufacturer's recommendations.

Checking resuscitation equipment following use

Checking of resuscitation equipment following use should be a specifically delegated responsibility. As well as the routine checks identified above, any disposable equipment used should be replaced and reusable equipment, e.g. self-inflating bag, cleaned following local infection control procedures and manufacturer's recommendations. Any difficulties with equipment encountered during resuscitation should be documented and reported to relevant personnel.

Chapter summary

This chapter has detailed what resuscitation equipment should be immediately available in the event of a cardiac arrest. Suggestions have been made regarding the storage, checking and maintenance of this equipment.

References

Resuscitation Council (UK) (2004) *Recommended Minimum Equipment for In-Hospital Adult Resuscitation.* http://www.resus.org.uk/pages/eqipIHAR.htm. Accessed 14 July 2008.

Resuscitation Council UK (2009) http://www.resus.org.uk/pages/eqipIHAR.htm. Accessed 23 April 2009.

Royal College of Anaesthetists, Royal College of Physicians of London, Intensive Care Society & Resuscitation Council (UK) (2008) *Cardiopulmonary Resuscitation: standards for clinical practice and training A Joint Statement from The Royal College of Anaesthetists, The Royal College of Physicians of London, The Intensive Care Society, The Resuscitation Council (UK).* The Royal College of Anaesthetists, London.

Chapter 3

Recognition and Treatment of the Critically Ill Patient

Introduction

Less than 20% of patients who have a cardiopulmonary arrest in hospital are discharged home (Nolan *et al.*, 2005). Critically ill patients have a high risk of cardiopulmonary arrest. Prompt recognition and early effective treatment of these patients may prevent further deterioration and maximise the chances of recovery (Gwinnutt, 2006). This proactive approach may negate the need for admission to the intensive care unit (ICU) and could reduce mortality and morbidity for those admitted at the appropriate time (McQuillan *et al.*, 1998; McGloin *et al.*, 1999; Young *et al.*, 2003).

The aim of this chapter is to understand the recognition and treatment of the critically ill patient.

Learning outcomes

At the end of this chapter the reader will be able to:

- Discuss the importance of prevention of in-hospital cardiopulmonary arrest
- List the clinical signs of critical illness
- Discuss the role of outreach and medical emergency teams
- Describe the assessment and emergency treatment of the critically ill patient

Prevention of in-hospital cardiopulmonary arrest

Survival to discharge from in-hospital cardiopulmonary arrest

In the UK, only 17% of patients who have an in-hospital cardiopulmonary arrest survive to discharge (Nolan *et al.*, 2005). Most of these survivors will have received prompt and effective defibrillation for a monitored and witnessed ventricular fibrillation arrest, caused by primary myocardial ischaemia (Resuscitation Council (UK), 2006b). Survival to discharge in these patients is very good, even as high as 42% (Gwinutt *et al.*, 2000).

Unfortunately, most in-hospital cardiopulmonary arrests are caused by either asystole or pulseless electrical activity (PEA), both non-shockable rhythms associated with a very poor outcome (Nolan *et al.*, 2005). These arrests are not usually sudden or unpredictable: cardiopulmonary arrest usually presents as a final step in a sequence of progressive deterioration of the presenting illness, involving hypoxia and hypotension (Resuscitation Council (UK), 2006b). These patients rarely survive to discharge; the only approach that is likely to be successful is prevention of the cardiopulmonary arrest (Gwinnutt, 2006). For this prevention strategy to be successful, recognition and effective treatment of patients at risk of cardiopulmonary arrest is paramount. This may prevent some cardiac arrests, deaths and unanticipated ICU admissions (Nolan *et al.*, 2005). The ACADEMIA study demonstrated that antecedents were present in 79% of cardiopulmonary arrests, 55% of deaths and 54% of unanticipated ICU admissions (Kause *et al.*, 2004).

Sub-optimal critical care

Studies have shown that the care of critically ill inpatients in the UK is frequently sub-optimal (McQuillan *et al.*, 1998; McGloin *et al.*, 1999). Junior staff frequently fail to recognise and appreciate the severity of illness and when therapeutic interventions are implemented these have often been delayed or are inappropriate. The management of deteriorating inpatients is a significant problem, particularly at night and at weekends, when responsibilities for these patients usually falls to the acute take team whose main focus is on a rising tide of new admissions (Baudouin & Evans, 2002).

In a confidential inquiry into quality of care before admission to the ICU, two external reviewers assessed the quality of care in 100 consecutive admissions to ICU (McQuillan *et al.*, 1998):

- 20 patients were deemed to have been well managed and 54 to have received sub-optimal management, with disagreement about the remainder
- Case mix and severity were similar between the groups, but ICU mortality was worse in those who both reviewers agreed received sub-optimal care (48% compared with 25% in the well managed group)
- Admission to the ICU was considered late in 37 patients in the sub-optimal group. Overall, a minimum of 4.5% and a maximum of 41% of admissions were considered potentially avoidable
- Sub-optimal care contributed to morbidity or mortality in most instances
- The main causes of sub-optimal care were failure of organisation, lack of knowledge, failure to appreciate clinical urgency, lack of supervision and failure to seek advice

Even more disturbingly, studies of events leading to 'unexpected' in-hospital cardiac arrest indicate that many patients have clearly recorded evidence of marked physiological deterioration prior to the event, without appropriate action being taken (Franklin & Mathew, 1994; Schein *et al.*, 1990).

Deficiencies in critical care frequently involve simple aspects of care, e.g. failure to recognise and effectively treat abnormalities of the patient's airway, breathing and circulation, incorrect use of oxygen therapy, failure to monitor the patient, failure to ask for help from senior colleagues, ineffective communication, lack of teamwork and failure to use treatment limitation plans (McQuillan *et al.*, 1998; Hodgetts *et al.*, 2002).

The ward nurse is uniquely based to recognise that the patient is starting to deteriorate and to alert the appropriate help (Adam & Osborne, 2005). However, response times by ward staff are unacceptably variable (Rich, 1999).

Strategies to prevent in-hospital cardiac arrest

Nolan *et al.* (2005) suggest that the following strategies may help to prevent avoidable in-hospital cardiopulmonary arrests:

- Provide care for patients who are critically ill or at risk of clinical deterioration in appropriate areas, with the level of care provided matched to the level of patient sickness
- Critically ill patients need regular observations: match the frequency and type of observations to the severity of illness or the likelihood of clinical deterioration and cardiopulmonary arrest. Often only simple vital sign observations (pulse, blood pressure, respiratory rate) are needed
- Use an early warning score (EWS) system to identify patients who are critically ill and/or at risk of clinical deterioration and cardiopulmonary arrest
- Use a patient charting system that enables the regular measurement and recording of EWSs
- Have a clear and specific policy that requires a clinical response to EWS systems. This should include advice on the further clinical management of the patient and the specific responsibilities of medical and nursing staff
- The hospital should have a clearly identified response to critical illness. This may include a designated outreach service or resuscitation team (e.g. medical emergency team (MET)) capable of responding to acute clinical crises identified by clinical triggers or other indicators. This service must be available 24 hours per day
- Train all clinical staff in the recognition, monitoring and management of the critically ill patient. Include advice on clinical management while awaiting the arrival of more experienced staff
- Identify patients for whom cardiopulmonary arrest is an anticipated terminal event and in whom CPR is inappropriate, and patients who do not wish to be treated with CPR. Hospitals should have a do not attempt resuscitation (DNAR) policy, based on national guidance, which is understood by all clinical staff
- Ensure accurate audit of cardiac arrest, 'false arrest', unexpected deaths and unanticipated ICU admissions using common datasets. Audit also the antecedents and clinical response to these events

Clinical signs of critical illness

The clinical signs of critical illness and deterioration are usually similar regardless of the underlying cause, because they reflect compromise of the respiratory, cardiovascular and neurological functions (Nolan *et al.*, 2005). These clinical signs are commonly:

- Tachypnoea
- Tachycardia
- Hypotension
- Altered conscious level (e.g. lethargy, confusion, restlessness or falling level of consciousness)
(Resuscitation Council (UK), 2006b)

Tachypnoea, a particularly important indicator of an at-risk patient (Goldhill *et al.*, 1999), is the most common abnormality found in critical illness (Goldhill & McNarry, 2004). Fieselmann *et al.* (1993) found that a raised respiratory rate (>27/minute) occurred in 54% of patients in the 72 hours preceding cardiac arrest, most of which occurred at 72 hours prior to the event.

The identification of abnormal clinical signs (together with the patient's history, examination and appropriate investigations) is central to objectively identifying patients who are at risk of deterioration (Buist *et al.*, 1999). However, these clinical signs of deterioration are often subtle and can go unnoticed. It is therefore essential that tools, which reflect best evidence, are developed and available to aid the practitioner to identify signs of deterioration. Ultimately this may prevent adverse events and improve patient outcomes.

Early warning scores and calling criteria

Many hospitals now use early warning scores (EWSs) or calling criteria systems to help in the early detection of critical illness (Goldhill *et al.*, 1999; Hodgetts *et al.*, 2002; Subbe *et al.*, 2003; Buist *et al.*, 2004). Their sensitivity, specificity and reliability to predict clinicaloutcomeshaveyettobeconvincinglyproven(Cutherbertson, 2003; Parr, 2004). However, there is a sound rationale for using these systems to identify sick patients early (Nolan *et al.*, 2005).

Although there is no data demonstrating the best system, the EWS approach may be preferable because it tracks changes in physiology and warns of impending physiological collapse, while the calling criteria approach is only triggered if an extreme physiological value is recorded (Nolan *et al.*, 2005).

Early warning scores

Comprehensive Critical Care (Department of Health, 2000) recommended the widespread implementation of EWS systems and outreach services. The EWS systems have been developed as a tool to enable ward staff to combine their regular observations to produce an aggregate physiological score (Sharpley & Holden, 2004). They are based upon the premise that there is a common physiological pathway of deterioration in the critically ill patient, which can be detected by simple ward-based observations (Goldhill, 2001).

A weighted score is attached to a combination of blood pressure, pulse, respiratory rate, oxygen saturations, temperature, urine output and simplified level of consciousness (AVPU); this is then recorded on the patient's EWS observation chart (Figure 3.1). Once a certain score is reached, nursing and other paramedical staff must then alert the designated expert help following local protocols. Escalation policies are put in place whereby a failure to improve (or to receive prompt help) results in the immediate contact of more senior members (including consultant staff) (Baudouin & Evans, 2002). Clear guidelines should be drawn up to guide the nurse when and whom to contact for help (Figure 3.2).

Each hospital should have a track and trigger system that allows rapid detection of the signs of early clinical deterioration and an early and appropriate response (National Confidential Enquiry into Patient Outcome and Death (NCEPOD), 2005; National Institute for Health and Clinical Excellence (NICE), 2007). These track and trigger systems should be robust, should cover all inpatients and should be linked to a response team that is appropriately skilled to assess and manage the clinical problems (NCEPOD, 2005). However, 27% of hospitals do not use an early warning system (NCEPOD, 2005).

The main advantages of EWS systems are:

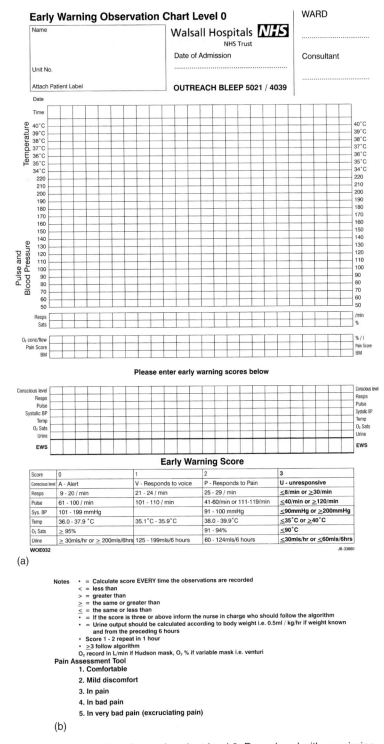

Early Warning Observation Chart Level 0

WARD

....

Name

Walsall Hospitals **NHS**
NHS Trust

Date of Admission

Consultant

Unit No.

....

Attach Patient Label

OUTREACH BLEEP 5021 / 4039

Please enter early warning scores below

Early Warning Score

Score	0	1	2	3
Conscious level	A - Alert	V - Responds to voice	P - Responds to Pain	U - unresponsive
Resps	9 - 20 / min	21 - 24 / min	25 - 29 / min	≤8/min or ≥30/min
Pulse	61 - 100 / min	101 - 110 / min	41-60/min or 111-119/min	≤40/min or ≥120/min
Sys. BP	101 - 199 mmHg		91 - 100 mmHg	≤90mmHg or ≥200mmHg
Temp	36.0 - 37.9 °C	35.1°C - 35.9°C	38.0 - 39.9°C	≤35°C or ≥40°C
O₂ Sats	≥ 95%		91 - 94%	≤90°C
Urine	≥ 30mls/hr or ≥ 200mls/6hrs	125 - 199mls/6 hours	60 - 124mls/6 hours	≤30mls/hr or ≤60mls/6hrs

WOE032

JB-33880

(a)

Notes
- = Calculate score EVERY time the observations are recorded
- < = less than
- > = greater than
- ≥ = the same or greater than
- ≤ = the same or less than
- = If the score is three or above inform the nurse in charge who should follow the algorithm
- = Urine output should be calculated according to body weight i.e. 0.5ml / kg/hr if weight known and from the preceding 6 hours
- Score 1 - 2 repeat in 1 hour
- ≥3 follow algorithm
- O₂ record in L/min if Hudson mask, O₂ % if variable mask i.e. venturi

Pain Assessment Tool
1. Comfortable
2. Mild discomfort
3. In pain
4. In bad pain
5. In very bad pain (excruciating pain)

(b)

Fig. 3.1 Early warning observation chart level 0. Reproduced with permission of Walsall Hospitals NHS Trust.

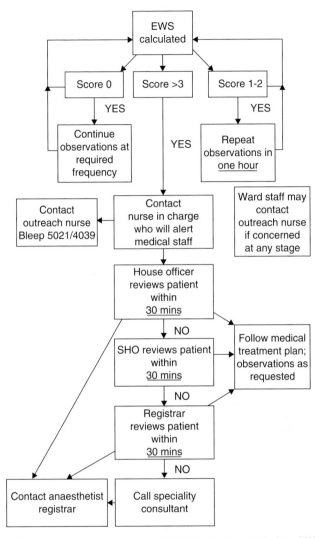

Fig. 3.2 Early warning score algorithm. Reproduced with permission of Walsall Hospitals NHS Trust.

- Simplicity: only the basic monitoring equipment is required (usually readily available on acute wards)
- Reproducibility between different observers
- Applicability to multi-professional team
- Minimal staff training required

(Gwinnutt, 2006)

Best practice – EWS:

- EWS score should be designed to reflect subtle changes in condition
- EWS chart should be straightforward to use and unambiguous in its design
- Implementation should be planned and coordinated
- Extensive education strategy prior to implementation
- Specific guidelines attached to the EWS, e.g. whom to call and when
- EWS calling criteria can be adjusted for specific patients, e.g. chronic disease
- Audit of EWS charts to assess completeness
- Audit of specific incidents where calling criteria were not adhered to
- Ongoing education of staff

Physiological track and trigger systems should be used to monitor all patients in acute hospital settings at least every 12 hours, unless:

- A decision is made by a senior member of the team to increase or decrease this frequency for a particular patient
- Abnormal physiology is detected – a graded response will be required (see below)

(NICE, 2007)

Graded-response strategy

A graded response strategy for patients who have been identified as being at risk of clinical deterioration should be agreed at a local level:

- *Low-score group*: increased frequency of observations and the nurse in charge informed
- *Medium-score group*: urgent call to the team primarily responsible for the care of the patient and to personnel with core competencies for treating acute illness, e.g. critical care outreach, hospital-at-night team

- *High-score group*: emergency call to a team with critical care competencies and diagnostic skills – should include a medical practitioner skilled in the assessment and treatment of the critically ill patient, who has advanced airway management and resuscitation skills; this should be an immediate response

(NICE, 2007)

Calling criteria systems

'Calling criteria' systems are based on routine observations, which activate a response when an extreme physiological value is reached (Lee *et al.*, 1995; Goldhill *et al.*, 1999).

Role of outreach and medical emergency teams

Outreach teams

Comprehensive Critical Care (Department of Health, 2000) recommended the development of outreach teams in all acute trusts. They have been established in accordance with the 'intensive care without walls' philosophy as one aspect of the critical care service (Gwinnutt, 2006). The objectives of outreach teams are to:

- Avert ICU admissions by identifying patients who are deteriorating and either helping to prevent admission or ensuring that admission to a critical care bed happens in a timely manner to ensure best outcome
- Enable ICU discharges by supporting both the continuing recovery of discharged patients on wards and after discharge from hospital
- Share critical care skills with staff in wards and the community, ensuring enhancement of training opportunities and skills practice and using information gathered from the ward and community to improve critical care services for patients and relatives

(Department of Health, 2000)

All acute trusts should have a formal outreach service that is available 24 hours per day, seven days per week (NCEPOD, 2005; NICE, 2007). The composition of this service will vary from hospital to hospital but it should comprise of individuals with the skills and ability to recognise and manage the problems of critical illness (NCEPOD, 2005). Outreach services should not replace the role of traditional medical teams in the care of inpatients, but should be seen as complementary (NCEPOD, 2005).

However, many outreach services are often not available on a 24-hour basis (NCEPOD, 2005). Some only provide cover for selected patients, e.g. postoperative surgery (NCEPOD, 2005); 44% of hospitals do not even provide an outreach service (NCEPOD, 2005).

Despite widespread acceptance of and intuitive belief in the benefit of outreach teams, there is a lack of evidence to support their use, there are national variations in their availability, there is no consensus about the ideal composition and there is no consensus regarding triggers to activate referral (Holder & Cuthbertson, 2005).

Best practice – outreach teams:

- Clear operational guidelines
- Structured work practices
- Ownership by senior trust managers and clinicians
- Clear lines of communication throughout the organisation
- Form strong links with other teams to share practice and disseminate ideas
- Identify and address training needs in ward areas
- Act as a resource and support for ward staff

Medical emergency teams

In some hospitals the cardiac arrest team, which has been traditionally only been called once the patient has had a cardiopulmonary arrest, has been replaced by a medical emergency team (MET) (Nolan *et al.*, 2005). The MET not only responds to patients in cardiopulmonary arrest, but also to those with acute physiological deterioration (Lee *et al.*, 1995). METs were first developed in Australia in the 1990s where they are now commonplace. The MET approach demonstrates proactive and pre-emptive management of the patient at risk. The aim of a MET is to pre-empt deterioration and prevent adverse events (Lee *et al.*, 1995; Goldhill *et al.*, 1999; Bristow *et al.*, 2000; Buist *et al.*, 2002; Bellomo *et al.*, 2003).

METs are reliant upon calling criteria, whereupon the team will automatically be called. They will then assess and treat the patient as required with the explicit aim of preventing deterioration. Evidence is currently emerging exploring the efficacy of METs and improvement in outcomes. Members of the MET may include:

- Experienced ICU nurse
- Anaesthetist
- Physician

Best practice – MET:

- Calling criteria should be evidence based
- Staff must be aware of the MET calling criteria
- MET calling criteria should be visible in all wards and departments
- Staff should carry individual copies of MET calling criteria
- Regular education sessions to update staff
- MET education sessions on all staff orientation programmes
- Audit of all MET calls to identify trends and deficiencies
- Audit of cardiac arrests
- Utilise data as part of learning needs analysis
- Inappropriate MET calls should be dealt with sensitively so that staff are not discouraged to call MET in the future

Assessment and emergency treatment of the critically ill patient

Safety

Ensure the environment is safe and free of hazards and follow infection control guidelines, e.g. wash hands, put on gloves if necessary.

Communication

Talk to the patient and evaluate his response: a normal response, indicates he has a clear airway, is breathing and has adequate cerebral perfusion; the inability to complete sentences could indicate extreme respiratory distress. An inappropriate response or no response could indicate an acute life-threatening physiological disturbance (Gwinnutt, 2006).

Patient's general appearance

Note the patient's general appearance, his colour and whether he appears content and relaxed or distressed and anxious.

Senior help

During the assessment process, consider whether senior help should be requested.

Oxygen

Administer high-concentration oxygen: attached oxygen 15 litres/minute to an oxygen mask with an oxygen reservoir (sometimes referred to as a non-rebreathe mask) (Figure 3.3).

Monitoring devices

Attach appropriate monitoring devices, e.g. pulse oximetry, electrocardiogram (ECG) monitor and non-invasive blood pressure monitoring, as soon as it is safe to do so (Resuscitation Council (UK), 2006b).

ABCDE assessment

The Resuscitation Council (UK) (2006b) has issued guidelines on the recognition and treatment of the critically ill patient. Adapted from the ALERT course (Smith, 2003), these guidelines follow the logical and systematic ABCDE approach to patient assessment:

- Airway
- Breathing
- Circulation
- Disability
- Exposure

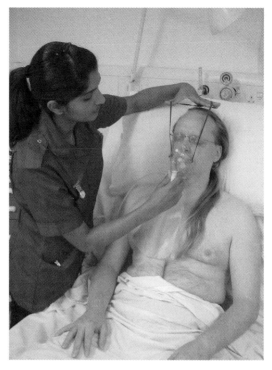

Fig. 3.3 Non-rebreathe mask to administer high-concentration oxygen.

When assessing the patient, undertake a complete initial assessment, identifying and treating life-threatening problems first, before moving onto the next part of assessment. The effectiveness of treatment/intervention should be evaluated, and regular reassessment undertaken. The need to alert more senior help should be recognised and other members of the multi-disciplinary team should be utilised as appropriate so that patient assessment, instigation of appropriate monitoring and interventions can be undertaken simultaneously.

Irrespective of their training, experience and expertise in clinical assessment and treatment, all nurses can follow the ABCDE approach; clinical skills, knowledge, expertise and local circumstances will determine what aspects of the assessment and treatment are undertaken.

Assessment of airway

Look, listen and feel for the signs of airway obstruction. Partial airway obstruction will result in noiy breathing:

- *Gurgling*: indicates the presence of fluid, e.g. secretions or vomit, in the mouth or upper airway; usually seen in a patient with altered conscious level who is having difficulty or is unable to clear his own airway
- *Snoring*: indicates that the pharynx is being partially obstructed by the tongue; usually seen in a patient with altered conscious level lying in a supine position
- *Stridor*: high-pitched sound during inspiration, indicating partial upper airway obstruction; usually due to either a foreign body or laryngeal oedema
- *Wheeze*: noisy musical whistling type sound due to the turbulent flow of air through narrowed bronchi and bronchioles, more pronounced on expiration; causes include asthma and chronic obstructive pulmonary disorder (COPD)

Complete airway obstruction can be detected by no air movement at the patient's mouth and nose. Paradoxical chest and abdominal movements ('see-saw' movement of the chest) may be observed and if not rapidly treated, central cyanosis will develop (a late sign of airway obstruction).

Treatment of an obstructed airway

> **Treat airway obstruction as a medical emergency and obtain expert help immediately. Untreated, airway obstruction leads to a lowered PaO_2 and risks hypoxic damage to the brain, kidneys and heart, cardiac arrest, and even death. (Resuscitation Council (UK), 2006b)**

- If the airway is compromised, treat the underlying cause, e.g. administer suction to the mouth if the patient has vomited, place the patient in the lateral position (unless contraindicated). The most common underlying cause of airway obstruction in hospital is altered conscious level leading to structures in the mouth, e.g. the tongue, to block the airway. In these patients, simple airway techniques can be very effective, e.g. head tilt, chin lift, use of an oropharyngeal airway. Occasionally, advanced airway techniques, e.g. tracheal intubation, may be needed.

- Administer high-concentration oxygen as soon as possible in a patient with an obstructed airway (Resuscitation Council UK, 2006b).

Assessment of breathing

Look, listen and feel to assess breathing.

Count the respiratory rate: normal respiratory rate is 12–20/minute (Resuscitation Council (UK), 2006b). Tachypnoea is usually first sign that the patient has respiratory distress (Smith, 2003). Bradypnoea is an ominous sign and could indicate imminent respiratory arrest; causes include drugs, e.g. opiates, fatigue, hypothermia, head injury and central nervous system (CNS) depression.

Evaluate chest movement: chest movement should be symmetrical; unilateral chest movement suggests unilateral pathology, e.g. pneumothorax, pneumonia, pleural effusion (Smith, 2003).

Evaluate depth of breathing: only marked degrees of hyperventilation and hypoventilation can be detected; hyperventilation may be seen in metabolic acidosis or anxiety and hypoventilation may be seen in opiate toxicity (Ford *et al.*, 2005).

Evaluate respiratory pattern: Cheyne-Stokes breathing pattern (periods of apnoea alternating with periods of hyperpnoea) can be associated with brain stem ischaemia, cerebral injury and severe left ventricular failure (altered carbon dioxide sensitivity of the respiratory centre) (Ford *et al.*, 2005).

Note the oxygen saturation (SaO_2) reading: normal is 97–100%. A low SaO_2 could indicate respiratory distress or compromise. N.B. the pulse oximeter does not detect hypercapnia and the SaO_2 can be normal in the presence of a very high $PaCO_2$ (Resuscitation Council (UK), 2006b).

Listen to the breathing: normal breathing is quiet. Rattling airway noises indicate the presence of airway secretions, usually due to patient being unable to cough sufficiently or unable to take a deep breath in (Smith, 2003). The presence of stridor or wheeze indicates partial, but significant, airway obstruction (see above).

Check the position of the trachea: place the tip of the index finger into the supersternal notch, let it slip either side of the trachea and determine whether it fits more easily into one or other side of the trachea (Ford *et al.*, 2005). Deviation of the trachea to one side indicates mediastinal shift (e.g. pneumothorax, lung fibrosis or pleural fluid).

Palpate the chest wall: to detect surgical emphysema or crepitus (suggesting a pneumothorax *until* proven otherwise) (Smith, 2003).

Perform chest percussion:

1. Place the left hand on the patient's chest wall. Ensure the fingers are slightly separated, with the middle finger pressed firmly into the intercostals space to be percussed (Ford *et al.*, 2005)
2. Strike the centre of the middle phalanx of the middle finger sharply using the tip of the middle finger of the right hand (Ford *et al.*, 2005) (Figure 3.4). Deliver the stroke using a quick flick of the wrist and finger joints, not from the arm or shoulder. The percussing finger should be bent so that its terminal phalanx is at right angles to the metacarpal bones when the blow is delivered, and it strikes the percussed finger in a perpendicular way. The percussing finger should then be removed immediately, like a clapper inside a bell, otherwise the resultant sound will be dampened (Epstein *et al.*, 2003)
3. Percuss the anterior and lateral chest wall. Percuss the from side to side, top to bottom, comparing both sides and looking for asymmetry
4. Categorise the percussion sounds (see below)
5. If an area of altered resonance is located, map out its boundaries by percussing from areas of normal to altered resonance (Ford *et al.*, 2005)

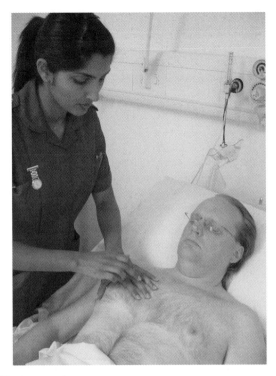

Fig. 3.4 Chest percussion.

6. Sit the patient forward and then percuss the posterior chest wall, omitting the areas covered by the scapulae. Ask the patient to move his elbows forward across the front of his chest: this will rotate the scapulae anteriorly and out of the way (Talley & O'Connor, 2001). It may be helpful to offer the patient a pillow to lean on
7. Again percuss from side to side, top to bottom, comparing both sides and looking for asymmetry. Don't forget that the lung extends much further down posteriorly than anteriorly (Epstein *et al.*, 2003)
8. Categorise the percussion sounds (see below)

Causes of different percussion notes (Ford *et al.*, 2005):

- Resonant: air-filled lung
- Dull: liver, spleen, heart, lung consolidation/collapse
- Stony dull: pleural effusion/thickening

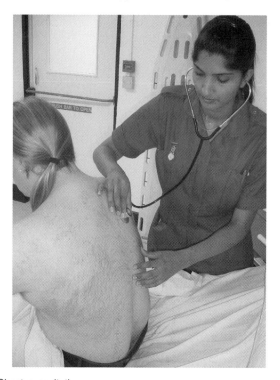

Fig. 3.5 Chest auscultation.

- Hyper-resonant: pneumothorax, emphysema
- Tympanitic: gas-filled viscus

Auscultate the chest (Figure 3.5):

1. Ask the patient to breath in and out normally through his mouth
2. Auscultate the anterior chest from side to side, and top to bottom. Auscultate over equivalent areas and compare the volume and character of the sounds and note any additional sounds. Compare the sounds during inspiration and expiration
3. Note the location and quality of the sounds heard
4. Auscultate the posterior chest, from side to side and top to bottom. Auscultate over equivalent areas and compare the volume and character of the sounds and note any additional

sounds. Compare the sounds during inspiration and expiration (Jevon & Cunnington, 2007)

Evaluate air entry, the depth of breathing and the equality of breath sounds on both sides of the chest. Bronchial breathing indicates lung consolidation; absent or reduced sounds suggest a pneumothorax or pleural fluid (Smith, 2003). In particular, note any additional breath sounds:

- *Wheezes (rhonchi)*: high-pitched musical sounds associated with air being forced through narrowed airways, e.g. asthma (Ford *et al.*, 2005). Usually more pronounced on expiration. Inspiratory wheeze (stridor) is usually indicative of severe upper airway obstruction, e.g. foreign body, laryngeal oedema. If both inspiratory and expiratory wheezes are heard, this is usually due to excessive airway secretions (Adam & Osborne, 2005)
- *Crackles (crepitations)*: non-musical sounds – associated with reopening of collapsed airway, e.g. pulmonary oedema (Ford *et al.*, 2005). Crackles are usually localised in pneumonia and mild cases of bronchiectasis; in pulmonary oedema and fibrosing alveolitis, both lung bases are equally affected (Epstein *et al.*, 2003)
- *Pleural friction rub*: leathery/creaking sounds during inspiration and expiration, evident in areas of inflammation when the normally smooth pleural surfaces are roughened and rub on each other (Adam & Osborne, 2005)

Record peak expiratory flow rate: provides a useful estimate of the calibre of the airways particularly in asthma and COPD (Ford *et al.*, 2005).

Evaluate efficacy of breathing, work of breathing & adequacy of ventilation:

- *Efficacy of breathing*: air entry, chest movement, pulse oximetry, arterial blood gas analysis and capnography
- *Work of breathing*: respiratory rate and accessory muscle use, e.g. neck and abdominal muscles
- *Adequacy of ventilation*: heart rate, skin colour and mental status

> If the patient has compromised breathing it is paramount to provide prompt effective treatment. In addition, during the initial assessment of breathing, it is essential to diagnose and effectively treat immediately life-threatening conditions, e.g. acute severe asthma, pulmonary oedema, tension pneumothorax, massive haemothorax (Resuscitation Council (UK), 2006b).

Treatment of compromised breathing
1. Ensure the patient has a clear airway
2. Ideally, sit the patient upright (to maximise chest movement)
3. Administer high concentration of oxygen via a non-rebreathe mask (Figure 3.3) (Jevon, 2007); if the patient has COPD, high concentrations of oxygen can lead to respiratory depression: in these patients aim for oxygen saturations of 90–92% (PaO$_2$ of 8 kPa or 60 mmHg) (Resuscitation Council (UK), 2006b). However, if a patient with COPD is acutely breathless, administer high concentrations of oxygen: the patient is more likely to suffer adverse effects from hypoxia than respiratory depression (Smith, 2003)
4. If possible, treat the underlying cause, e.g. administer nebulised salbutamol in a patient having a severe asthma attack
5. If the patient's breathing is inadequate, start ventilation

Assessment of circulation

Look, listen and feel to assess circulation.

Palpate peripheral and central pulses: assess presence, rate, quality, regularity and equality (Smith, 2003). A weak thready pulse suggests a poor cardiac output and bounding pulse may indicate sepsis (Resuscitation Council (UK), 2006b).

Check the colour and temperature of the hands and fingers: signs of cardiovascular compromise include cool and pale peripheries.

Measure the capillary refill time (CRT): apply sufficient pressure to cause blanching to the skin, e.g. sternum, for 5 seconds and then release. Normal CRT is <2 seconds; a prolonged CRT could indicate poor peripheral perfusion, though other causes can include cool ambient temperature, poor lighting and old age (Resuscitation Council (UK), 2006b).

Look for other signs of a poor cardiac output: e.g. altered conscious level and, if the patient has a urinary catheter, oliguria (urine volume <0.5 ml/kg/hour) (Smith, 2003).

Look for signs of haemorrhage: e.g. from wounds or drains or evidence of internal haemorrhage, e.g. abdominal swelling; concealed blood loss can be significant, even if drains are empty (Smith, 2003).

Measure blood pressure (BP): systolic BP < 90 mmHg suggests shock. A normal BP does not exclude shock because compensatory mechanisms increase peripheral resistance in response to reduced cardiac output (Smith, 2003). A low diastolic BP suggests arterial vasodilatation, e.g. anaphylaxis or sepsis. A narrowed pulse pressure, i.e. the difference between systolic and diastolic readings (normal is 35–45 mmHg), suggests arterial vasoconstriction, e.g. cardiogenic shock or hypovolaemia (Resuscitation Council (UK), 2006b).

Assess the state of the veins: if hypovolaemia is present the veins could be under-filled or collapsed (Smith, 2003)

Interpret the ECG: determine whether a cardiac arrhythmia is present. A 12-lead ECG should he recorded as a priority in some situations, e.g. chest pain.

Treatment of shock

In almost all medical and surgical emergencies, if the patient is hypotensive, hypovolaemia should be considered to be the primary cause of shock, until proven otherwise (Resuscitation Council (UK), 2006b).

1. Ensure the patient has a clear airway and adequate breathing

2. Administer high concentration of oxygen via a mask with a non-rebreathe bag
3. Lie the patient flat, ideally with the bottom of the bed raised
4. Insert one or more large wide-bore intravenous cannulae (14 or 16 gauge); take bloods, e.g. fullblood count (FBC), cross-match if necessary, administer fluid challenge, e.g. 500 ml of 0.9% saline stat (1000 mls if the patient is hypotensive; 250 ml if the patient has confirmed heart failure – auscultate the chest for crepitations after each bolus) (Resuscitation Council (UK), 2006a)
5. Repeat the fluid challenge if the patient does not improve
6. Treat the underlying cause of shock and ensure expert help is called

Treatment of acute coronary syndrome
1. Assess the patient following the ABCDE approach
2. Call for help
3. Record a 12-lead ECG
4. Treatment includes oxygen, aspirin, glyceryl trinitrate spray, morphine and reperfusion therapy (see Chapter 11)

Assessment of disability

Assess disability (CNS function):

- *Evaluate the patient's level of consciousness*: use AVPU (Figure 3.6) or the Glasgow Coma Scale (GCS) if a more objective assessment of conscious level is required, e.g. head injury
- *Examine the pupils*: compare size, equality and reaction to light of each pupil

A = **A**lert   V = Responds to **v**oice (speech)   P = Responds to **p**ainful stimuli   U = **U**nresponsive to any stimulus

Fig. 3.6 The AVPU scale to evaluate level of consciousness. Reproduced with permission from Resuscitation Council (UK).

Treatment of altered conscious level
1. Ensure the patient has a clear airway, adequate breathing and circulation
2. Administer high-concentration oxygen
3. Ideally nurse the patient in the lateral position
4. Check the patient's medication chart for reversible drug-induced cause of altered conscious level and administer appropriate antagonist, e.g. nalaxone for opiate overdose (Resuscitation Council (UK), 2006a)
5. Correct hypoglycaemia: e.g. administer 50 ml of 10% glucose IV (Resuscitation Council (UK), 2006a)
6. Call for help early

Exposure

Expose the patient and undertake a thorough examination to ensure important details are not over-looked (Smith, 2003). In particular, the examination should concentrate on the part of the body which is most likely contributing to the patient's ill status, e.g. in suspected anaphylaxis, examine the skin for urticaria. Respect the patient's dignity and minimize heat loss. In addition:

- Take a full clinical history and review the patient's notes/charts
- Study the recorded vital signs: trends are more significant than one-off recordings
- Administer prescribed medications
- Review laboratory results and ECG and radiological investigations
    Ascertain what level of care the patient requires (e.g. ward, high-dependency unit (HDU), ICU).
- Document in the patient's notes details of assessment, treatment and response to treatment.

(Resuscitation Council (UK), 2006b)

Chapter summary

Critically ill patients have a high morbidity and high mortality. Prognosis following an in-hospital cardiopulmonary arrest is poor. Prompt recognition and early appropriate management of critically ill patients are essential to prevent deterioration. Track and trigger systems should be in place to identify at-risk patients and alert expert help.

References

Adam S, Osborne S (2005) *Critical Care Nursing Science and Practice*, 2nd Ed. Oxford University Press, Oxford.

Baudouin S, Evans T (2002) Improving outcomes for severely ill medical patients. Editorial. *Clinical Medicine* (March/April)

Bellomo R, Goldsmith D, Shigehiko U *et al.* (2003) A prospective before and after trial of a medical emergency team. *Medical Journal of Australia* **179**(6):283–7.

Bristow PJ, Hillman KM, Chey T *et al.* (2000) Rates of in-hospital arrests, deaths and intensive care admissions: the effect of the medical emergency team. *Medical Journal of Australia* **173**:236–40.

Buist M, Jarmolowski E, Burton P *et al.* (1999) Recognising clinical instability in hospital patients before cardiac arrest or unplanned admission to intensive care. *Medical Journal of Australia* **171**:22–5.

Buist M, Moore G, Bernard S *et al.* (2002) Effects of a medical emergency team on reduction of incidence of and mortality from unexpected cardiac arrests in hospital: preliminary study. *British Medical Journal* **324**:1–5.

Buist M, Bernard S, Nguyen TV *et al.* (2004) Association between clinically abnormal observations and subsequent in-hospital mortality: a prospective study. *Resuscitation* **62**:137–41.

Cutherbertson B (2003) Outreach critical care – cash for no questions? *British Journal of Anaesthesia* **90**(1):5–6.

Department of Health (2000) *Comprehensive Critical Care*. Department of Health, London.

Epstein O, Perkin G, Cookson J, de Bono D (2003) *Clinical Examination*, 3rd Ed. Mosby, London.

Fieselmann JF, Hendryx MS, Helms CM *et al.* (1993) Respiratory rate predicts cardiopulmonary arrest for internal medicine patients. *Journal of General Internal Medicine* **8**:354–60.

Ford M, Hennessey I, Japp A (2005) *Introduction to Clinical Examination*. Elsevier, Oxford.

Franklin C, Mathew J (1994) Developing strategies to prevent in-hospital cardiac arrest: analyzing responses of physicians and nurses in the hours before the event. *Critical Care Medicine* **22**:244–7.

Goldhill DR, Worthington L, Mulcahy A *et al.* (1999) The patient-at-risk team: identifying and managing seriously ill patients. *Anaesthesia* **54**:853–60.

Goldhill D (2001) The critically ill: following your MEWS. *QJM* **94**:507–10.

Goldhill D, McNarry A (2004) Physiological abnormalities in early warning scores are related to mortality in adult inpatients. *British Journal of Anaesthesia* **92**(6):882–4.

Gwinutt CL, Columb M, Harris R (2000) Outcome after cardiac arrest in adults in UK hospitals: effect of the 1997 guidelines. *Resuscitation* **47**:125–35.

Gwinnutt C (2006) *Clinical Anaesthesia*, 2nd Ed. Blackwell Publishing, Oxford.

Hodgetts TJ, Kenward G, Vlackonikolis I *et al.* (2002) Incidence, location and reasons for avoidable in-hospital cardiac arrest in a district general hospital. *Resuscitation* **54**:115–23.

Holder P, Cuthbertson B (2005) Critical care without the intensive care unit. *Clinical Medicine* **5**:449–51.

Jevon P (2007) Respiratory procedures part 1: use of a non-rebreathing oxygen mask. *Nursing Times* **103**(32):26–7.

Jevon P, Cunnington A (2007) Cardiovascular examination part 3: auscultation of the heart. *Nursing Times* **103**(27):24–5.

Kause J, Smith G, Prytherch D *et al.* (2004) A comparison of antecedents to cardiac arrests, deaths and emergency intensive care admissions in Australia and New Zealand, and the United Kingdom – the ACADEMIA study. *Resuscitation* **62**:275–82.

Lee A, Bishop G, Hillman K, Daffurn K (1995) The Medical Emergency Team. *Anaesthesia and Intensive Care* **23**:183–6.

McGloin H, Adam SK *et al.* (1999) Unexpected deaths and referrals to intensive care of patients on general wards. Are some cases potentially preventable? *Journal of the Royal College of Physicians* **33**(3):255–9.

McQuillan P, Pilkington S, Allan A *et al.* (1998) Confidential enquiry into quality of care before admission to intensive care. *British Medical Journal* **316**:1853–8.

National Confidential Enquiry into Patient Outcome and Death (2005) *An Acute Problem?* NCEPOD, London.

National Institute for Health and Clinical Excellence (2007) *Acutely Ill Patients in Hospital: Recognition of and Response to Acute Illness in Adults in Hospital.* NICE, London.

Nolan J, Deakin C, Soar J *et al.* (2005) European Resuscitation Council Guidelines for Resuscitation 2005: Section 4. Adult advanced life support. *Resuscitation* **675S**:S39–S86.

Parr M (2004) Critical care outreach: some answers, more questions. *Intensive Care Medicine* **30**:1261–2.

Resuscitation Council (UK) (2006a) *Immediate Life Support*, 2nd Ed. Resuscitation Council (UK), London.

Resuscitation Council (UK) (2006b) *Advanced Life Support*, 5th Ed. Resuscitation Council (UK), London.

Rich K (1999) In-hospital cardiac arrest: pre-event variables and nursing response. *Clinical Nurse Specialist* 147–53.

Schein RMH, Hazday N, Pena M *et al.* (1990) Clinical antecedents to in-hospital cardiac arrest. *Chest* **98**:1388–92.

Sharpley JT, Holden JC (2004) Introducing and early warning scoring system in a district general hospital. *Nursing in Critical Care* **9**(3): 98–103.

Smith AF, Wood J (1998) Can some in-hospital cardio-respiratory arrests be prevented? *Resuscitation* **37**:133–7.

Smith G (2003) ALERT Acute Life-Threatening Events Recognition and Treatment, 2nd Edn. University of Portsmouth, Portsmouth.

Subbe CP, Davies RG, Williams E *et al.* (2003) Effect of introducing the modified early warning score on clinical outcomes, cardio-pulmonary arrests and intensive care utilisation in acute medical admissions. *Anaesthesia* **58**:775–803.

Talley N, O'Connor S (2001) *Clinical Examination*, 4th Ed. Blackwell Publishing, Oxford.

Young MP, Gooder VJ, McBride K *et al.* (2003) Inpatient transfers to the Intensive Care Unit. *Journal of General Internal Medicine* **18**:77–83.

Chapter 4

Principles of Cardiac Monitoring and ECG Recognition

Introduction

Cardiac monitoring forms an integral part of cardiopulmonary resuscitation (CPR). Once the presenting electrocardiogram (ECG) rhythm has been identified, the appropriate treatment can then be administered. Poor technique can lead to an inaccurate ECG trace and mistaken diagnosis; a sound knowledge of the principles of cardiac monitoring is essential.

An understanding of the principles of ECG recognition is also important. It will enable the identification of abnormal ECG rhythms which may compromise cardiac output, precede or be associated with cardiac arrest, or complicate recovery after successful CPR.

The aim of this chapter is to understand the principles of cardiac monitoring and ECG recognition.

Learning outcomes

At the end of this chapter the reader will be able to:

- Describe the conduction system of the heart
- Describe the ECG and its relation to cardiac contraction
- List three methods of cardiac monitoring
- State the problems that can be encountered with cardiac monitoring
- Outline a systematic approach to ECG interpretation
- Recognise cardiac arrhythmias associated with cardiac arrest
- Recognise peri-arrest arrhythmias

The conduction system of the heart

The heart possesses specialised muscle cells that initiate and conduct electrical impulses resulting in myocardial contraction. The conduction system (Figure 4.1) comprises of the following:

- Sinus node (sinoatrial or SA node)
- Atrioventricular (AV) node or junction
- Bundle of His
- Bundle branches (right and left)
- Purkinje fibres

Nervous control of the heart rate

The sinus node normally acts as the pacemaker for myocardial contraction. The rate it fires is dependent upon the autonomic nervous system:

- *Parasympathetic or vagus nerve* – an increase in activity slows down the heart rate while a decrease in activity speeds up the

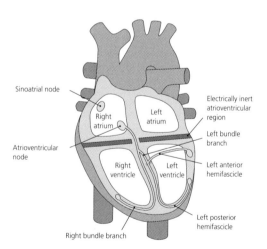

Fig. 4.1 The conduction system of the hear. Reproduced from Meek, S. & Morris, F. (2008) Introduction. I – leads, rate, rhythm, and cardiac axis. In: Morris, F., Brady, W. & Camm, J. (Eds) *ABC of Clinical Electrocardiography*, p. 1. Reprinted with permission from Wiley-Blackwell.

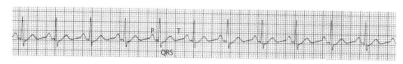

Fig. 4.2 The ECG and its relation to cardiac contraction.

heart rate. Atropine blocks the vagus nerve causing an increase in heart rate

- *Sympathetic nerve* – prepares the body for 'fight and flight' and will result in an increase in heart rate and an increase in the force of myocardial contraction. Beta blockers shield the heart from sympathetic nerve stimulation, resulting in a fall in heart rate and blood pressure and a reduction in myocardial workload

The ECG and its relation to cardiac contraction

1. The sinus node fires and the electrical impulse spreads across the atria causing atrial contraction (P wave) (Figure 4.2)
2. On arriving at the AV junction, the impulse is slowed to allow the atria time to fully contract and eject blood into the ventricles. This brief period of absent electrical activity is represented on the ECG by a straight (isoelectric) line between the end of the P wave and the beginning of the QRS complex
3. The impulse is then conducted to the ventricles through the bundle of His, right and left bundle branches and Purkinje fibres causing ventricular depolarisation and contraction (QRS complex)
4. The ventricles then repolarise (T wave)

(Jevon, 2002)

Methods of cardiac monitoring

Standard ECG leads

During CPR, lead II is recommended for cardiac monitoring (Resuscitation Council (UK), 2006). Lead II should be selected on

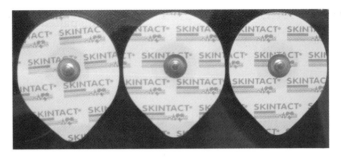

Fig. 4.3 ECG monitoring: ECG electrodes.

the monitor and the ECG electrodes (Figure 4.3) should be positioned as follows:

- *Red* on the right shoulder
- *Yellow* on the left shoulder
- *Green* on the left upper abdominal wall

This standard position for ECG electrode placement benefits from reduced muscle interference and will not hinder paddle placement for defibrillation.

Defibrillator paddles

Most modern manual defibrillators allow cardiac monitoring using the defibrillator paddles. This 'quick look' method enables rapid recognition of a shockable rhythm and prompt defibrillation.

'Paddle monitoring' should be selected on the defibrillator and gel pads used to ensure good contact. The paddles should be firmly applied to the gel pads on the chest, one just to the right of the sternum below the right clavicle and the other in the mid-axillary line, approximately level with the V6 electrode position (Resuscitation Council (UK), 2006). Applying the paddles according to their namesake will result in an upright lead II ECG trace, though for defibrillation this is not important.

The theoretical advantage of this method of cardiac monitoring is that it facilitates prompt recognition of ventricular fibrillation (VF) and subsequent defibrillation. In practice, however, the ECG trace may not be very clear and may be unreliable (spurious asystole) (Chamberlain, 1999). It is important to keep the paddles very still and not to interrupt chest compressions for any longer than a few seconds while assessing the ECG rhythm; cardiac monitoring should be established as soon as possible (Resuscitation Council (UK), 2006).

Large adhesive multifunctional electrodes

Automatic defibrillators and advisory defibrillators use large adhesive multifunctional electrodes which enable cardiac monitoring and defibrillation (some also allow external pacing). This method of cardiac monitoring and hands-free defibrillation during CPR is becoming more popular (Bradbury *et al.*, 2000).

The electrodes are applied to the patient's bare chest. The skin should be dry and it is sometimes necessary to quickly shave the patient's chest to ensure adequate skin contact. The standard position for the electrodes is the same as for defibrillator paddles described above. It is important to adhere to the manufacturer's recommendations when applying the electrodes and attaching the leads. If the patient has a permanent pacemaker device situated below the right clavicle, the anterior/posterior electrode position is recommended (Resuscitation Council (UK), 2006).

Problems encountered with cardiac monitoring

Problems encountered with cardiac monitoring include:

- *'Straight line' ECG trace* – check the patient, monitoring lead selected (normally lead II), ECG gain, ECG leads and electrodes. N.B. asystole is rarely a straight line
- *Poor quality ECG trace* – check all the connections and brightness display. Ensure the electrodes are correctly attached, are 'in-date' and that the gel sponge is moist, not dry (Perez, 1996). Ensure the skin where the electrodes are attached is dry. Wiping the skin with an alcohol wipe may help if problems persist. If the patient is sweating profusely the application of a small amount of tincture benzoin to the skin, leaving it to dry before applying the electrodes, is recommended (Jowett & Thompson, 1995)

- *Interference and artefacts* – poor electrode contact, patient movement, CPR and electrical interference, e.g. from bedside infusion pumps, can cause the ECG trace to be 'fuzzy'. Apply the electrodes over bone rather than muscle to minimise interference (Resuscitation Council (UK), 2006)
- *Wandering baseline* – ECG trace going up and down is usually caused by patient movement or simply by ventilation. Reposition the electrodes away from the lower ribs (Meltzer *et al.*, 1983)
- *Small ECG complexes* – causes of small and unrecognisable ECG complexes include pericardial effusion, obesity and hypothyroidism. It could be a technical problem; check that the ECG gain is adequate and the appropriate ECG monitoring lead is selected
- *Incorrect heart rate display* – causes include small QRS complexes, large T waves, muscle movement and interference. Ensure the ECG trace is adequate

Systematic approach to ECG interpretation

To accurately interpret an ECG trace requires considerable experience and expertise. However it is possible to interpret most ECG traces and arrive at a reliable diagnosis on which to base effective treatment, by following a systematic approach to ECG interpretation:

- Is electrical activity present?
- What is the QRS rate?
- Is the QRS rhythm regular or irregular?
- Is the QRS complex width normal or broad?
- Are P waves present?
- How are P waves related to QRS complexes?

(Resuscitation Council (UK), 2006)

Is electrical activity present?

If there is no electrical activity check the gain control (ECG size), ECG leads, ECG electrodes, all electrical connections and the defibrillator/cardiac monitor ensuring it is switched on. If there is no electrical activity and the patient is pulseless, the diagnosis is asystole (Resuscitation Council (UK), 2006). The line is usually distorted due to drift of the baseline, electrical interference and CPR. Sometimes P waves may be present indicating 'P wave asystole' or ventricular standstill.

A completely straight line is usually caused by disconnection of ECG leads or wrong monitoring lead, e.g. 'paddles' selected on the defibrillator when monitoring with ECG leads. If electrical activity is present, ascertain whether there are any recognisable ECG complexes. If there aren't any, VF is the probable diagnosis. If recognisable ECG complexes can be identified the following five steps should be followed.

What is the QRS rate?

Estimate the QRS rate by counting the number of large (1 cm) squares between two adjacent QRS complexes and dividing it into 300, e.g. the QRS rate in Figure 4.4 is about 85 (300/3.5). Care should be taken if the QRS rate is irregular.

- Normal ventricular rate is 60–100
- Bradycardia is <60
- Tachycardia is >100

Is the QRS rhythm regular or irregular?

Establish whether the QRS rhythm is regular or irregular by carefully comparing the R-R intervals at different sections on the ECG rhythm strip. If the QRS rhythm is irregular, ascertain whether it is totally irregular, e.g. in atrial fibrillation, or whether there is a cyclical pattern to the irregularity, e.g. extrasystoles, pauses, dropped beats, where the relationship between the P waves and QRS complexes is particularly important (see below).

Is the QRS complex width normal or broad?

Note the width of the QRS complex. The normal width is less than three small squares (0.12 seconds). If the width of the QRS complex is broad (three small squares or more), the rhythm may be ventricular in origin or supraventricular in origin, but

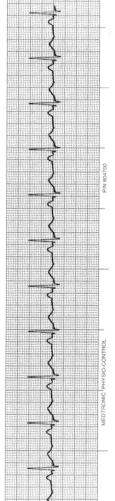

Fig. 4.4 Sinus rhythm.

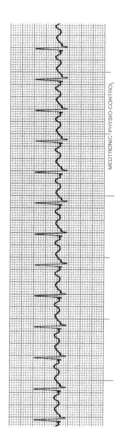

Fig. 4.5 Sinus tachycardia.

transmitted with aberrant conduction. A broad complex tachycardia is most likely to be ventricular in origin.

Are P waves present?

Establish whether P waves are present and calculate the rate and regularity. Sometimes it can be difficult or even impossible to determine whether P waves are present because they can be partially or totally obscured by QRS complexes and T waves.

How are P waves related to QRS complexes?

If P waves are present, ascertain whether each one is followed by a QRS complex and whether each QRS complex is preceded by a P wave. Calculate the PR interval; the normal range is three to five small squares (0.12–0.20 seconds). A shortened or prolonged PR interval is indicative of a conduction abnormality. If the PR interval is constant it is probable that atrial and ventricular activity are related.

If the PR interval is variable, establish whether there is a pattern to the variability. Plot out the P waves and QRS complexes and look for any recognisable pattern between the two, the occurrence of missed or dropped beats and PR intervals that vary in a repeated fashion. Complete dissociation between atrial and ventricular activity may be indicative of third-degree complete AV block.

Sinus rhythm (Figure 4.4)

- *QRS rate* – 60–100
- *QRS rhythm* – regular
- *QRS width* – normal
- *P waves* – present, normal
- *Relationship between P waves and QRS complexes* – P wave precedes each QRS complex

Sinus rhythm is the normal rhythm of the heart. The impulse originates in the sinus node at a rate of 60–100 beats/min, is regular and is conducted down the normal pathways and with no abnormal delays. Sometimes sinus rhythm without a pulse (pulseless electrical activity) can be seen during a cardiac arrest.

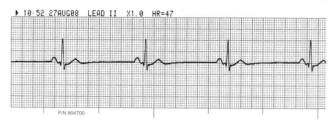

Fig. 4.6 Sinus bradycardia.

Sinus tachycardia (Figure 4.5)

- *QRS rate* – >100
- *QRS rhythm* – regular
- *QRS width* – normal
- *P waves* – present, normal but >100
- *Relationship between P waves and QRS complexes* – P wave precedes each QRS complex

Sinus bradycardia (Figure 4.6)

- *QRS rate* – <60
- *QRS rhythm* – regular
- *QRS width* – normal
- *P waves* – present, normal but < 60
- *Relationship between P waves and QRS complexes* – P wave precedes each QRS complex

Cardiac arrhythmias associated with cardiac arrest

Ventricular fibrillation

All coordination of electrical activity in the ventricular myocardium is lost, resulting in loss of cardiac output and cardiac arrest. The ECG is characteristic, showing a bizarre irregular waveform which is apparently random in both amplitude and frequency (Figure 4.7). It can be classified as either coarse or fine. Fine ventricular fibrillation can sometimes be mistaken for asystole, hence the importance of ensuring the ECG gain is adequate. The definitive treatment is early defibrillation.

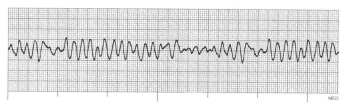

Fig. 4.7 Ventricular fibrillation.

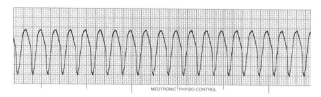

Fig. 4.8 Broad complex tachycardia.

Broad complex tachycardia (Figure 4.8)

- *QRS rate* – 100–300, usually about 180
- *QRS rhythm* – regular
- *QRS width* – broad (0.12 seconds or more)
- *P waves* – may be identifiable
- *Relationship between P waves and QRS complexes* – if able to identify P waves there is AV dissociation

Broad complex tachycardia usually results from a focus in the ventricles firing at a rapid rate. The patient may or may not lose cardiac output. The ECG configuration can vary depending on where in the ventricles the focus is. In the event of cardiac arrest the definitive treatment is early defibrillation.

Asystole

Although asystole is often referred to as a 'straight line', in reality it is represented by an undulating line (Figure 4.9). In all cases of apparent asystole, the ECG trace should be viewed with suspicion before arriving at a final diagnosis. Other causes of a straight line ECG trace should be excluded, e.g. incorrect lead setting,

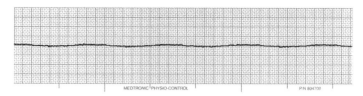

Fig. 4.9 Asystole.

disconnected leads and inadequate ECG gain. Sometimes p waves are present – ventricular standstill or ventricular asystole.

Pulseless electrical activity (Figure 4.4)

Pulseless electrical activity (PEA) does not refer to a specific ECG rhythm; it defines a clinical situation where there is no cardiac output despite the presence of an ECG trace that would normally be expected to produce one (Resuscitation Council (UK), 2006).

Peri-arrest arrhythmias

Peri-arrest arrhythmias can be defined as malignant arrhythmias that may lead to cardiac arrest or complicate the post-resuscitation period (Colquhoun & Vincent, 2004). They are defined according to the heart rate as this will dictate the initial treatment (Resuscitation Council (UK), 2006).

Bradyarrhythmia

A bradyarrhythmia can be defined as a ventricular (QRS) rate <60 per minute (Resuscitation Council (UK), 2006); a pathological bradyarrhythmia can be caused by a disturbance in impulse formation or conduction. In some patients it can be a normal finding.

First-degree AV block (Figure 4.10)
- *QRS rate* – usually approximately 60–80
- *QRS rhythm* – regular
- *QRS width* – normal

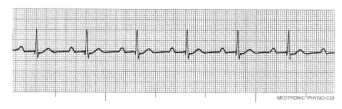

Fig. 4.10 First-degree AV block.

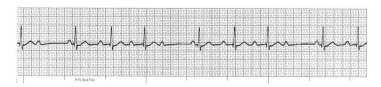

Fig. 4.11 Second-degree AV block Mobitz type I (Wenkebach).

- *P waves* – present, normal
- *Relationship between P waves and QRS complexes* – P wave precedes each QRS complex, but PR interval prolonged to more than five small squares

First-degree AV block is characterised by a prolonged PR interval. Usually no treatment is required. If there is a new development, cardiac monitoring is required to detect any progression to second- or third-degree blocks.

Second-degree AV block Mobitz type I (Wenkebach) (Figure 4.11)

- *QRS rate* – usually 60–80
- *QRS rhythm* – irregular
- *QRS width* – normal
- *P waves* – present and normal
- *Relationship between P waves and QRS complexes* – not every P wave is followed by a QRS complex; there is gradual prolonging of the PR interval

Second-degree AV block Mobitz type I (Wenkebach) is characterised by the progressive prolonging of the PR interval until the

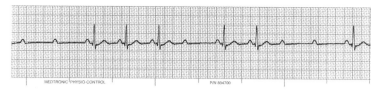

Fig. 4.12 Second-degree AV block Mobitz type II.

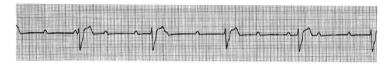

Fig. 4.13 Third-degree (complete) AV block.

conduction of the impulse to the ventricles does not occur and a beat is dropped. Caused by a delay in the AV junction, it is usually benign.

Second-degree AV block Mobitz type II (Figure 4.12)

- *QRS rate* – usually 50–70
- *QRS rhythm* – irregular
- *QRS width* – normal
- *P waves* – present, normal
- *Relationship between P waves and QRS complexes* – not every P wave is followed by a QRS complex. PR interval in conducted beats is constant.

Second-degree AV block Mobitz type II is a serious cardiac arrhythmia that can degenerate to third-degree atrioventricular block or ventricular standstill. Cardiac pacing is usually required.

Third-degree (complete) AV block (Figure 4.13)

- *QRS rate* – usually 30–50
- *QRS rhythm* – regular
- *QRS width* – broad (0.12 seconds or more)
- *P waves* – present, normal
- *Relationship between P waves and QRS complexes* – AV dissociation

In third-degree or complete atrioventricular block, impulses from the atria are blocked and do not reach the ventricles. The atria and ventricles continue to beat at their intrinsic rate and there is atrioventricular dissociation. Third-degree heart block can degenerate into ventricular standstill and cardiac arrest.

Tachyarrhythmias

Tachyarrhythmias are classified as either narrow complex tachycardia (originating above the ventricles, i.e. in the atria or AV junction) or broad complex tachycardia (usually originating in the ventricles, i.e. below the AV junction) (Colquhoun & Vincent, 2004).

Narrow complex tachycardia (Figure 4.14)
- *QRS rate* – usually 150–200
- *QRS rhythm* – regular
- *QRS width* – normal
- *P waves* – usually unidentifiable
- *Relationship between P waves and QRS complexes* – not applicable

Narrow complex tachycardia (formally termed supraventricular tachycardia or SVT) originates from above the bifurcation of the bundle of His. A 12-lead ECG will help confirm whether it is atrial or junctional in origin.

Atrial fibrillation (Figure 4.15)
- *QRS rate* – variable
- *QRS rhythm* – irregular and erratic
- *QRS width* – normal

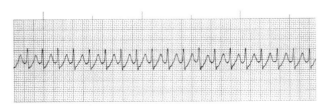

Fig. 4.14 Narrow complex tachycardia.

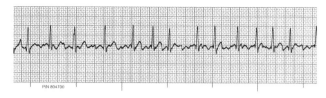

Fig. 4.15 Atrial fibrillation.

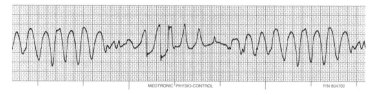

Fig. 4.16 Torsades de pointes.

- *P waves* – none identifiable, baseline is irregular and chaotic
- *Relationship between P waves and QRS complexes* – not applicable

Atrial fibrillation, characterised by totally disorganised electrical activity in the atria, is the most common cardiac arrhythmia encountered in clinical practice (Resuscitation Council (UK), 2006). An irregular QRS rhythm, absent P waves and a chaotic baseline are classical ECG features.

Torsades de pointes (Figure 4.16)

Torsades de pointes is characterised by 'twisting of the points' in which the axis of the electrical activity changes in a rotational way (Resuscitation Council (UK), 2006). It can degenerate into VF and cardiac arrest.

Chapter summary

The conduction system of the heart and the ECG and its relation to cardiac contraction have been described. Methods of cardiac monitoring, together with problems that can be encountered have been discussed. A systematic approach to ECG interpretation has been outlined, together with the recognition of important cardiac arrhythmias.

References

Bradbury N, Hyde D, Nolan J (2000) Reliability of ECG monitoring with a gel pad/paddle combination after defibrillation. *Resuscitation* **44**: 203–206.

Chamberlain D (1999) Spurious asystole with use of manual defibrillators. *British Medical Journal* **319**:1574.

Colquhoun M, Vincent R (2004) Management of peri-arrest arrhythmias. In: Colquhoun M *et al.* (Eds) *ABC of Resuscitation*, 5th Ed. Blackwell Publishing, Oxford.

Jevon P (2002) *ECGs for Nurses*. Blackwell Publishing, Oxford

Jowett N, Thompson D (1995) *Comprehensive Coronary Care*, 2nd Ed. Scutari Press, London

Meltzer LE, Pinneo R, Kitchell JR (1983) *Intensive Coronary Care, A Manual for Nurses*, 4th Ed. Prentice-Hall, London.

Perez A (1996) Cardiac monitoring: mastering the essentials. *Registered Nurse* **59**(8):32–9.

Resuscitation Council (UK) (2006) *Advanced Life Support Manual*, 5th Ed. Resuscitation Council (UK), London.

Chapter 5

Bystander Basic Life Support

Introduction

The term basic life support (BLS) refers to maintaining an open airway and supporting breathing and circulation without the use of equipment other than a protective shield (Handley *et al.*, 2005). A key component in the chain of survival (see Chapter 1), BLS is one of only two interventions that have been shown unequivocally to improve long-term survival following a cardiac arrest, the other being early defibrillation (Resuscitation Council (UK), 2006).

There are 700 000 deaths in Europe each year due to sudden cardiac arrest (Sans *et al.*, 1997). In many of these cases, ventricular tachycardia or ventricular fibrillation will be the initial arrhythmia: effective bystander BLS will increase the chances of survival, buying time while awaiting the arrival of the defibrillator.

Nurses need to have a working knowledge of BLS in case they need to perform it outside their normal working environment as a bystander or if they are teaching a lay person how to perform it.

The aim of this chapter is to understand the principles of bystander BLS.

Learning outcomes

At the end of the chapter the reader will be able to:

- Outline the potential hazards when attempting bystander BLS
- Discuss the initial assessment and sequence of actions in BLS
- Describe the principles of chest compressions

- Describe the principles of mouth-to-mouth ventilation
- Outline the treatment for foreign body airway obstruction

Potential hazards when attempting BLS

Nurses should eliminate, or at least minimise, any potential hazards associated with attempting bystander BLS. Potential hazards could include the environment, poisoning and infection. In addition national guidelines for safer handling during cardio-pulmonary resuscitation (CPR) should be followed (Resuscitation Council (UK), 2001).

Environment

Although unlikely to be a problem in the hospital setting, environmental hazards to BLS could include traffic, electricity, gas etc.

Poisoning

The casualty's exhaled air should be avoided in hydrogen cyanide or hydrogen sulphide gas poisoning. Ventilation should be undertaken using a non-return valve system.

Corrosive chemicals, e.g. strong acids, alkalis or paraquat, can easily be absorbed through the skin and respiratory tract; care should be taken when handling the casualty's clothes and bodily fluids, particularly vomit (Resuscitation Council (UK), 2006). Protective clothing and gloves should be worn.

Infection

Mouth-to-mouth ventilation is aesthetically unpleasant and rescuers are often reluctant to perform it even though the risk of cross-infection is minimal (Nolan *et al.*, 2005). There have only been isolated reports of transmission of infection following mouth-to mouth ventilation (Handley *et al.*, 2005). None of these have involved human immunodeficiency virus (HIV) or hepatitis B virus. However, as blood remains the single most important source of the transmission of HIV and hepatitis B virus, there is a theoretical risk of their transmission during mouth-to-mouth ventilation in cases of facial trauma, or if there are breaks in the skin around the lips or soft tissues of the oral cavity mucosa. Caution is particularly warranted in these situations.

Universal precautions also apply to blood, semen, vaginal secretions and cerebrospinal, synovial, pleural, peritoneal, pericardial and amniotic fluids and any body fluid containing visible blood (Centers for Disease Control, 1988). Care with sharps is paramount as both HIV and the hepatitis B virus have been contracted by healthcare workers following needle-stick injuries (Marcus, 1988).

Toxic gases or substances

If the casualty has been exposed to toxic gases, e.g. hydrogen cyanide, ventilation must be provided with a mask with a non-return valve so that the rescuer is not exposed to the casualty's exhaled air (Resuscitation Council (UK), 2006). Particular care should also be taken if the casualty has been exposed to toxic chemicals.

Problems associated with moving and handling

There are potential problems associated with moving and handling during resuscitation. Guidelines from the Resuscitation Council (UK) (2001) on safer handling during resuscitation should be observed to reduce the risk of self-injury:

- Assess the situation
- Adopt a position close to and directly facing the patient
- Avoid twisting the back
- Keep the spine in a neutral position
- Face the patient straight on

Initial assessment and sequence of actions in bystander BLS

The initial assessment and sequence of actions in bystander BLS outside the healthcare environment are outlined below, based on the Resuscitation Council (UK) algorithm for adult BLS (Figure

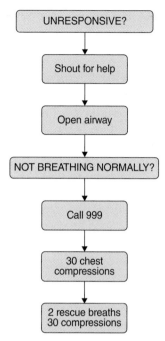

Fig. 5.1 Adult basic life support algorithm. Reproduced with permission of Resuscitation Council (UK).

5.1). On finding a collapsed, apparently lifeless casualty, ensure it is safe to approach and then check responsiveness.

Safety

Ensure there are no hazards (see above) and it is safe to approach. Proceed to ascertain whether the casualty is unresponsive.

Unresponsive?

Gently shake the casualty's shoulders and ask loudly, 'Are you all right?'

Responsive: leave the casualty in the position in which he has been found, provided there is no further danger. Establish the likely cause of the collapse and get help if necessary.

No response: shout out for help.

Shout for help

Shout for help; a bystander's assistance may be required, e.g. to alert the emergency services, to fetch an automated external defibrillator (AED) or to assist with CPR. Proceed to open the airway.

Open airway

Turn the casualty on to his back (unless full assessment is possible in the position in which he has been found). Open the airway by tilting the head and lifting the chin (Figure 5.2) (caution if cervical spine injury suspected). Proceed to ascertain whether the casualty is not breathing normally.

Not breathing normally?

While maintaining an open airway, ascertain for no longer than 10 seconds whether the casualty is breathing normally:

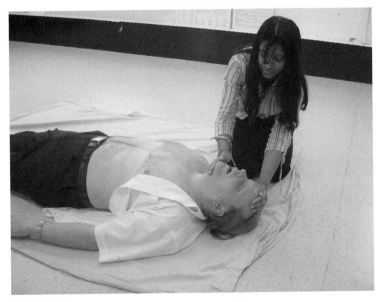

Fig. 5.2 Open the airway by tilting the head and lifting the chin.

- Look for chest movements
- Listen for airflow at the mouth and nose
- Feel for airflow on your cheek

During the first few minutes following a cardiac arrest, agonal breathing (infrequent noisy gasps) may be evident; do not confuse this with normal breathing (Resuscitation Council (UK), 2006).

Casualty breathing normally: place in the recovery position (see below), check for continued breathing and ensure the emergency services are alerted.

Casualty not breathing normally: call 999.

Call 999

It is important to ensure that the emergency services are immediately alerted. Ask a bystander to call 999 (Figure 5.3); a lone rescuer will need to do this first before starting chest compressions. Proceed to 30 chest compressions.

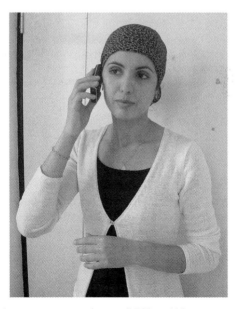

Fig. 5.3 Alert the emergency services: call 999 or 112.

30 chest compressions

Perform 30 chest compressions at a rate of 100 per minute (just under 2 per second). After 30 compressions, deliver two rescue breaths.

Two rescue breaths, 30 compressions

Deliver two rescue breaths, followed by 30 compressions. If unable or unwilling to deliver rescue breaths, perform chest compressions only at a rate of 100 per minute (see compression-only CPR section below) (Handley *et al.*, 2005). If there is more than one person present who can perform CPR, rotate them every 1–2 minutes to avoid fatigue.

Continue CPR until help arrives. The rescuer should only stop CPR if:

- Qualified help arrives and takes over
- The casualty begins to breathe normally
- Exhausted

(Handley *et al.*, 2005)

Principles of chest compressions

Related physiology

Chest compressions produce circulatory blood flow by increasing intrathoracic pressure and by directly compressing the heart (Handley *et al.*, 2005). Although effective chest compressions still only achieve systolic blood pressures of between 60 and 80 mmHg (Paradis *et al.*, 1989), this is still sufficient to maintain adequate coronary and cerebral blood flow, thus optimising the chance of successful defibrillation (Handley *et al.*, 2005). A palpable carotid or femoral pulse is not a reliable indicator of effective arterial blood flow during chest compressions (Ochoa *et al.*, 1997). Unfortunately chest compression technique is often poor (Abella *et al.*, 2005).

Following a break in chest compressions, the systolic blood pressure plummets and several chest compressions are then required to reach the pre-stoppage coronary and cerebral blood flow (Kern *et al.*, 1998). During resuscitation unnecessary and lengthy interruptions to chest compressions are frequent (Abella *et al.*, 2005) and efforts should be made to minimise these (Resuscitation Council (UK), 2005).

Procedure

1. Following confirmation of cardiac arrest, ask a bystander to call 999 (Figure 5.3) and, if appropriate, to fetch the automated external defibrillator, while starting chest compressions immediately
2. Ensure the casualty is supine on a firm flat surface, kneel in the high-kneeling position, at the side of the casualty level with his chest, with the knees shoulder-width apart (Resuscitation Council (UK), 2001)
3. Place the one hand on the centre of the casualty's chest (this equates to the middle of the lower half of the sternum) and then place the other on top (this is a quicker than wasting time using the 'rib margin' location method); do not apply pressure over the end of the sternum or the upper abdomen (Handley *et al.*, 2005)
4. To avoid applying pressure over the casualty's ribs, interlock and extend the fingers (Figure 5.4). Pressure should only be applied to the sternum and no pressure should be applied to the ribs, the end of the sternum or the upper abdomen (Handley *et al.*, 2005)
5. Position the shoulders directly vertical above the casualty's sternum, straighten the arms and lock the elbows (Figure 5.5); ensure the back is not twisted
6. Compress the sternum 4–5 cm (in adults) and, following each compression, allow the chest to completely recoil back to its normal position (Yannopoulos *et al.*, 2005), thus facilitating venous return. The force of compression should result from flexing the hips; the shoulders should be positioned directly above the casualty's sternum (Resuscitation Council (UK), 2001) – this will facilitate downward pressure
7. Perform chest compressions in a controlled manner; they should not be erratic or jerky (Jevon, 2006)
8. Continue chest compressions at a rate of 100/minute (Yu *et al.*, 2002); this rate refers to the speed of compressions rather than the actual number delivered per minute; interruptions

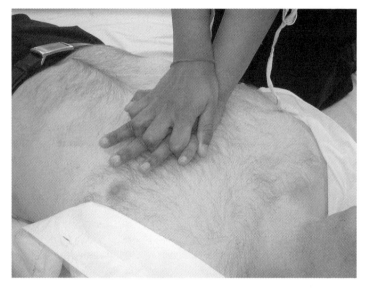

Fig. 5.4 Chest compressions: interlock the fingers.

in chest compressions, e.g. to allow defibrillation, will result in less than 100 being delivered in a minute

9. Ensure that the chest compression/chest relaxation phases are of equal duration
10. Ensure a ratio of 30 compressions: 2 ventilations (30:2) to allow more time for chest compressions
11. To prevent fatigue, rotate the person performing chest compressions approximately every 2 minutes (Nolan *et al.*, 2005)
12. Consider over-the-head chest compressions if the casualty is in a confined space
13. If unable or unwilling to perform mouth-to-mouth ventilation, perform chest compressions only at a rate of 100 per minute

(Jevon, 2006; Resuscitation Council (UK), 2006)

Chest compressions-only CPR

The American Heart Association (AHA) published a statement on compression-only CPR aimed at increasing the rate of

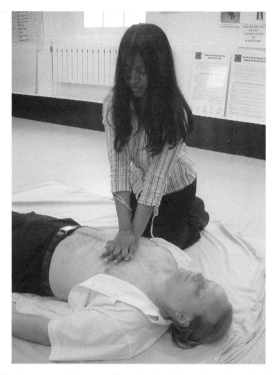

Fig. 5.5 Chest compressions: position the shoulders directly vertical above the patient's sternum, straighten the arms and lock the elbows.

bystander CPR and long-term survival following out-of-hospital cardiac arrest (Sayre *et al.*, 2008). The Resuscitation Council (UK) has endorsed this statement (Resuscitation Council (UK), 2008), reiterating their previously published guidance stating 'if you are not able, or are unwilling, to give rescue breaths, give chest compressions only' (Resuscitation Council (UK), 2006).

Principles of mouth-to-mouth ventilation

Mouth-to-mouth ventilation is a quick, effective way to provide adequate oxygenation and ventilation in a casualty who is not breathing (Wenzel *et al.*, 1994). However particular attention to the correct technique is essential. The most common cause of failure to ventilate is improper positioning of the head and chin (Idris *et al.*, 1996).

Barrier devices

Both healthcare workers and laypersons are often reluctant to perform mouth-to-mouth ventilation, usually due to a fear of contracting HIV (Resuscitation Council (UK), 2008). Consequently there is a variety of barrier devices available (Figure 5.6); face-masks with one-way valves prevent the transmission of bacteria, while face shields are less effective (Centers for Disease Control, 1991).

Procedure for mouth-to-mouth ventilation

1. Ensure the patient is supine. In a cardiac arrest, 30 chest compressions should have been performed first before delivering two ventilations (ratio 30:2) (Handley *et al.*, 2005)

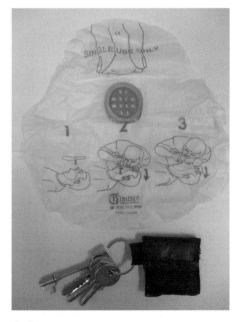

Fig. 5.6 Barrier device.

2. Kneel in a comfortable position with the knees shoulder-width apart, at the side of the patient at the level of his nose and mouth (a wider base will be required to undertake compressions if only one person is performing CPR) (Resuscitation Council (UK), 2001)
3. Rest back to sit on the heels in the low kneeling position (Resuscitation Council (UK), 2001)
4. Apply a barrier device if one is available and if trained in its use (Figure 5.6)
5. Bend forwards from the hips leaning down towards the patient's nose and mouth (Resuscitation Council (UK), 2001)
6. While maintaining head tilt and chin lift, pinch the soft part of the casualty's nose (use the index finger and thumb of the hand on the casualty's forehead), open the casualty's mouth and take a normal breath in (Figure 5.7)

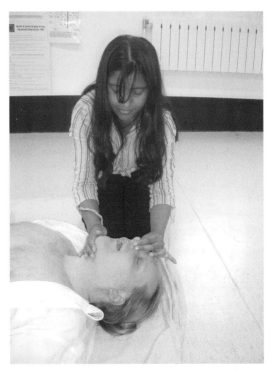

Fig. 5.7 Mouth-to-mouth ventilation: ensure an open airway and pinch the nose.

7. Place your lips around the casualty's mouth, ensuring a good seal, and blow into the casualty's mouth over 1 second and watch for chest rise
8. While still maintaining head tilt and chin lift, remove your mouth and watch for chest fall. Repeat the procedure and then ensure 30 chest compressions are performed
9. If the initial ventilation does not achieve chest rise as in normal breathing, before the next attempt, check the casualty's mouth and remove any obstruction and recheck to ensure adequate head tilt and chin lift and ensure adequate seal. Only attempt two ventilations before 30 chest compressions are performed again (Handley *et al.*, 2005)
10. If the casualty is on a bed: stand at the side facing the patient, level with his nose and mouth and bend forwards from the hips to minimise flexion of the spine; the nurse's weight can also be supported by resting the elbows on the bed and leaning the legs against the side of the bed frame (Resuscitation Council (UK), 2001)

(Jevon, 2006a; Resuscitation Council UK, 2006)

Ineffective delivery of rescue breaths

If it difficult to deliver effective breaths:

- Ensure adequate head tilt and chin lift
- Check the casualty's mouth and remove any obstruction
- Ensure a good seal between your mouth and the casualty's mouth
- Ensure the casualty's nose is pinched during ventilation

Minimising gastric inflation

Gastric inflation is commonly associated with mouth-to-mouth ventilation, occurring when the pressure in the oesophagus exceeds the opening pressure of the lower oesophageal sphincter pressure, resulting in the sphincter opening (Basket *et al.*, 1996). During CPR, the oesophageal sphincter relaxes, thus increasing the likelihood of gastric inflation (Bowman *et al.*, 1995). Complications of gastric inflation are detailed in Chapter 6.

Excessive tidal volumes or inspiratory flows can generate excessive airway pressures, which can lead to gastric inflation and the subsequent risk of regurgitation and aspiration of gastric contents (Nolan *et al.*, 2005). It is therefore recommended to deliver each ventilation over 1 second, with sufficient volume to achieve chest rise, but avoiding rapid and forceful ventilations (Handley *et al.*, 2005).

The recovery position

In an unconscious casualty the airway is at risk. Regurgitated gastric contents, debris in the mouth or upper airway, loose dentures or mechanical obstruction arising from structures in the mouth, e.g. the tongue and epiglottis, can all compromise the airway (Quinn, 1998).

The recovery position is designed to maintain a patent airway and reduce the risk of airway obstruction and aspiration (American Heart Association, 2005). It is advocated for most unconscious casualties. In the post-arrest situation, if the casualty is breathing spontaneously and does not require any further resuscitation, then appropriate positioning of the casualty using the recommended recovery position promotes the maintenance of a clear airway and helps prevent vomit or secretions from obstructing the airway and potentially causing aspiration.

The recovery position is also recommended in many other situations where the casualty's conscious level is compromised, e.g. following a major seizure (Bingham, 2004; Hayes, 2004) and during a hypoglycaemic coma (Diebel, 1999).

Spine injury

If the casualty has a known or suspected spinal injury, he should only be moved if an open airway cannot otherwise be maintained. Ideally the patient should be kept still in the position he is found, while awaiting the arrival of the emergency services. However, if it is necessary to move the casualty, e.g. compromised airway, the patient should ideally be carefully log-rolled, with the head and neck kept as still as possible and in alignment. Extension of the lower arm above the head together with bending both legs, while rolling the head on to the arm, may be feasible (American Heart Association, 2005).

Right or left lateral

Historically the left lateral position has been advocated for the recovery position (Eastwick-Field, 1996). However, there appear to be no cardiac autonomic tone advantages to be gained by placing a person in the recovery position one side compared with the other (Ryan *et al.*, 2003). Although either side can be used, in practical terms the environment can dictate which side is used, e.g. if the casualty has collapsed next to a wall, he will have to be rolled away from it.

Variations

There are several different variations of the recovery position, each with its own advantages (Handley *et al.*, 2005). However, no single technique is perfect for all patients (Handley, 1993; Turner *et al.*, 1997). The position used should be stable, near a true lateral position with the head dependent and no pressure applied to the chest which could impair breathing (American Heart Association, 2005).

Procedure

1. Check the environment and decide which is the best side to roll the casualty. Remove any obstacles if necessary
2. If necessary, remove the casualty's spectacles and place them in a safe place. Some authorities also recommend checking in the casualty's pockets and removing any sharp instruments, e.g. keys. If doing this proceed with extreme caution
3. Loosen any clothing around the neck
4. Kneel beside the casualty. To minimise the risk of self-injury, adopt a stable base with the knees shoulder-width apart, avoid twisting the back and keep the spine in a neutral position (Resuscitation Council (UK), 2001)
5. Ensure that both of his legs are straight
6. Position the arm nearest to the nurse perpendicular to the casualty's body with the elbow bent and the hand palm uppermost (Figure 5.8)

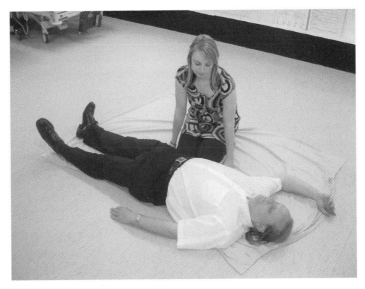

Fig. 5.8 Recovery position: position the arm nearest to the nurse perpendicular to the casualty's body with the elbow bent and the hand palm uppermost.

7. Grasp the far arm and bring it across the casualty's chest and hold the back of the hand against his cheek
8. Using the free hand, grasp the far leg just above the knee and pull it up, taking care to keep the patient's foot on the ground (Figure 5.9)
9. Whilst holding the casualty's hand against his cheek, pull on the far leg to roll the patient towards you on to his side
10. Adjust the casualty's upper leg, ensuring that both the hip and the knee are bent at right angles
11. Tilt the casualty's head back to ensure that the airway remains open
12. If necessary, adjust the hand under the patient's cheek to maintain the head tilted (Figure 5.10)
13. Monitor the casualty's vital signs

(Handley *et al.*, 2005; Jevon, 2006b; Resuscitation Council (UK), 2006)

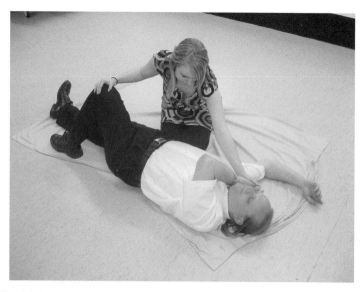

Fig. 5.9 Recovery position: using the free hand, grasp the far leg just above the knee and pull it up, taking care to keep the patient's foot on the ground.

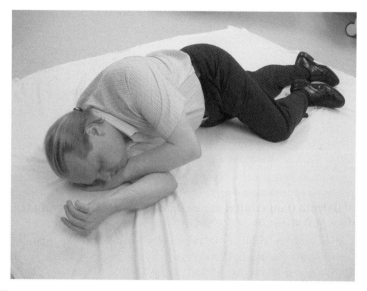

Fig. 5.10 Recovery position.

Complications

Even if the casualty is in the recovery position, airway, breathing and circulation can still become compromised. Closely monitor the casualty's vitals signs, particularly breathing (Handley *et al.*, 2005).

It has been reported that when the lower arm is placed in front, compression of vessels and nerves in the dependent limb can occur (Fulstow & Smith, 1993; Turner *et al.*, 1997). Therefore, monitor for signs of impaired blood flow in the lowermost arm (Rathgeber *et al.*, 1996) and ensure that the duration for which there is pressure on this arm is kept to a minimum (Resuscitation Council (UK), 2006). If the casualty needs to remain in the recovery position for longer than 30 minutes, turn him to the opposite side to relieve the pressure on the forearm (Handley *et al.*, 2005).

Treatment for foreign body airway obstruction

Foreign body airway obstruction (FBAO) (choking) is a life-threatening emergency. As most FBAO events are associated with eating, they are commonly witnessed, thus providing an opportunity for early intervention while the patient is still conscious (Handley *et al.*, 2005). Case reports have demonstrated the effectiveness of back blows, abdominal thrusts and chest thrusts for the treatment of FBAO (International Liaison Committee on Resuscitation (ILCOR), 2005), successful treatment often requiring more than one particular intervention.

Incidence

FBAO is an uncommon, yet potentially treatable, cause of accidental death (Fingerhut *et al.*, 1998). Each year in the UK approximately 16 000 adults and children receive treatment in A&E for FBAO (Handley *et al.*, 2005); less than 1% of these are fatal (Department of Trade & Industry, 1999). In adults the commonest cause of FBAO is food, e.g. meat, poultry and fish (Department of Trade & Industry, 1999); in children half of the cases are caused by food (usually sweets) and half are caused by such items as toys, coins etc. (Department of Trade & Industry, 1999a).

Recognition of FBAO

Complete FBAO is often characterised by a sudden inability to talk, maximal respiratory effort, development of cyanosis and clutching of the neck. In partial airway obstruction, the casualty will be distressed, may cough and may have a wheeze. In complete airway obstruction, the casualty will be unable to speak, breathe or cough and will eventually collapse and go unconscious. Always ask the casualty "Are you choking?" (Handley *et al.*, 2005). If he responds 'yes' by nodding his head without speaking, this indicates severe airway obstruction requiring urgent treatment (American Heart Association, 2005).

- If the casualty is choking, but able to breathe, encourage him to cough.
- If the casualty is choking but is unable to breathe or is displaying signs of becoming weak or stops breathing or coughing, immediate intervention is required.

Procedure

1. Stand at side, slightly behind the casualty
2. Support his chest with one hand and lean him well forward. This will help ensure that if the foreign body is dislodged, it will drop out of the mouth instead of slipping further down the airway
3. Deliver up to five back blows between the scapulae using the heel of the hand (Figure 5.11). After each back blow, check to see if it has been successful at relieving the obstruction
4. If the back blows fail, proceed to abdominal thrusts
5. Stand behind the casualty, placing both arms around his upper abdomen
6. Lean the casualty forward
7. Place a clenched fist between the casualty's umbilicus and xiphisternum and clasp it with the other hand (Figure 5.12)
8. Deliver up to five sharp thrusts to the abdomen, inwards and upwards
9. If the obstruction remains, continue alternating five back blows with five abdominal thrusts

(Resuscitation Council UK, 2006; Jevon, 2007)

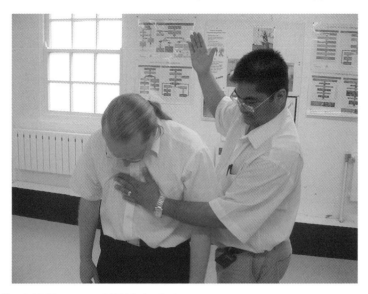

Fig. 5.11 Treatment of FBAO: back slap.

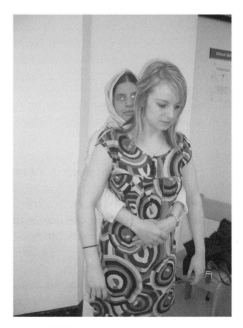

Fig. 5.12 Treatment of FBAO: abdominal thrust.

If the casualty loses consciousness:

- Carefully support him to the ground
- Immediately call 999
- Start CPR, 30 chest compressions first (even if there is a pulse) – chest compressions may relieve the obstruction

(Handley *et al.*, 2005)

Chest thrusts vs. abdominal thrusts

Chest thrusts can generate higher airway pressures than abdominal thrusts (Guildner *et al.*, 1976; Ruben & Macnaughton, 1978). If a patient with a FBAO loses consciousness, as chest thrusts are almost identical to chest compressions, CPR should be started (Handley *et al.*, 2005). Then each time the airway is opened to provide ventilations, check the mouth in case the foreign body has been dislodged.

Finger sweeps

The routine use of a finger sweep to clear the airway in the absence of visible airway obstruction has yet to be evaluated (Elam *et al.*, 1960; Hartrey & Bingham, 1995). Finger sweeps have been reported to have caused harm to both the casualty and the rescuer (ILCOR, 2005). Blind finger sweeps are not recommended; only manually remove a foreign body in the airway if it can be seen (Handley *et al.*, 2005).

Follow-up

Following successful treatment for a FBAO, a foreign body may still be present in the airways: therefore if the casualty has dysphagia, has a persistent cough or complains of having something 'stuck in his throat', he should be referred to a doctor (Handley *et al.*, 2005).

As abdominal thrusts can cause serious internal injury, e.g. rupture or laceration of abdominal or thoracic viscera, a casualty who has been treated with them must be referred to a doctor (ILCOR, 2005).

Chapter summary

Effective bystander BLS will help maintain an adequate circulation and ventilation until action can be taken to reverse the underlying cause of the cardiac arrest. It is often only a holding procedure, buying time while the means of reversing the underlying cause of the arrest can be obtained. Safe handling procedures should always be followed during CPR.

References

Abella B, Alvarado J, Myklebust H *et al.* (2005) Quality of cardiopulmonary resuscitation during in-hospital cardiac arrest. *Journal of the American Medical Association* **293**:305–10.

American Heart Association (2005) 2005 American Heart Association guidelines for cardiopulmonary resuscitation and emergency cardiovascular care. *Circulation* **112**:24 suppl.

Basket P, Nolan J, Parr M (1996) Tidal volumes which are perceived to be adequate for resuscitation. *Resuscitation* **3**:231–4.

Bingham E (2004) Epilepsy: diagnosis and support for people with epilepsy. *Practice Nursing* **15**(2):64–70.

Bowman F, Menegazzi J, Check B, Ducket T (1995) Lower esophageal sphincter pressure during prolonged cardiac arrest and resuscitation. *Annals of Emergency Medicine* **26**:216–9.

Centers for Disease Control (1988) Update: universal precautions for prevention of transmission of human immunodeficiency virus, hepatitis B virus and other blood-bourne pathogens in healthcare settings. *MMWR. Morbidity and Mortality Weekly Report* **37**:377–88.

Centers for Disease Control (1991) Nosocomial transmission of multi-drug-resistant tuberculosis among HIV-infected persons – Florida and New York. *MMWR. Morbidity and Mortality Weekly Report* **40**:585–91.

Department of Trade & Industry (1999) Choking. In: *Home and Leisure Accident Report*. Department of Trade & Industry, London

Department of Trade & Industry (1999a) *Choking Risks for Children*. Department of Trade & Industry, London

Diebel G (1999) The management of hypoglycaemia in type1 and type 2 diabetes. *British Journal of Community Nursing* **4**(9):454–60.

Eastwick-Field P (1996) Resuscitation: basic life support. *Nursing Standard* **10**(34):49–56.

Elam J, Ruben A, Greene D (1960) Resuscitation of drowning victims. *Journal of the American Medical Association* **174**:13–6.

Fingerhut L, Cox C, Warner M (1998) International comparative analysis of injury mortality. Findings from the ICE on injury statistics. International collaborative effort on injury statistics. *Advance Data* **12**:1–20.

Fulstow R, Smith G (1993) The new recovery position, a cautionary tale. *Resuscitation* **26**:89–91.

Guildner C, Williams D, Subitch T (1976) Airway obstructed by foreign material: the Heimlich maneuver. *JACEP* **5**:675–7.

Handley A (1993) Recovery position. *Resuscitation* **26**:93–5.

Handley A, Koster R, Monsieurs K *et al.* (2005) European Resuscitation Council Guidelines for Resuscitation 2005: Section 2. Adult basic life support and use of automated external defibrillators. *Resuscitation* **67S1**:S7-S23

Hartrey R, Bingham R (1995) Pharyngeal trauma as a result of blind finger sweeps in the choking child. *Journal of Accident & Emergency Medicine* **12**:52–4.

Hayes C (2004) Clinical skills: practical guide for managing adults with epilepsy. *British Journal of Nursing* **13**(7):380–7.

Idris AH, Florete OG Jr, Melker RJ *et al.* (1996) Physiology of ventilation, oxygenation and carbon dioxide elimination during cardiac arrest. In: Paradis NA, Halperin HR, Nowak RM (eds) *Cardiac Arrest: The Science and Practice of Resuscitation Medicine*. Williams & Wilkins, London.

International Liaison Committee on Resuscitation (ILCOR) (2005) Part 2 Adult basic life support 2005 international consensus on cardiopulmonary resuscitation and emergency cardiovascular care science with treatment recommendations. *Resuscitation* **67**:187–200.

Jevon P (2006) Cardiopulmonary resuscitation: chest compressions. *Nursing Times* **98**(22):47–8.

Jevon P (2006a) Mouth to mouth ventilation. *Nursing Times* **102**(37): 30–1.

Jevon P (2006b) Resuscitation skills-part 1: the recovery position. *Nursing Times* **102**(37):30–1

Jevon P (2007) Treatment for airway obstruction. *Nursing Times* **103**(9): 26–7.

Marcus R (1988) Surveillance of health care workers exposed to blood from patients infected with the human immunodeficiency virus. *New England Journal of Medicine* **319**:1118–23.

Nolan J, Deakin C, Soar J *et al.* (2005) European Resuscitation Council Guidelines for Resuscitation 2005: Section 4. Adult advanced life support. *Resuscitation* **675S**:S39-S86.

Ochoa F, Ramalle-Gomara E, Carpintero J *et al.* (1997) Competence of health professionals to check the carotid pulse. *Resuscitation* **37**:173–5.

Paradis N, Martin G, Goetting M *et al.* (1989) Simultaneous aortic, jugular bulb, and right atrial pressures during cardiopulmonary resuscitation in humans. Insights into mechanisms. *Circulation* **80**: 361–8.

Quinn T (1998) Cardiopulmonary resuscitation: new European guidelines. *British Journal of Nursing* **7**(18):1070–7.

Rathgeber J, Panzer W, Gunther U *et al.* (1996) Influence of different types of recovery positions on perfusion indices of the forearm. *Resuscitation* **32**:13–17.

Resuscitation Council (UK) (2001) *Guidance for Safer Handling During Resuscitation in Hospitals*. Resuscitation Council (UK), London.

Resuscitation Council (UK) (2005) *Guidelines 2005*. Resuscitation Council (UK), London.

Resuscitation Council (UK) (2006) *Advanced Life Support*, 5th Ed. Resuscitation Council (UK), London.

Resuscitation Council (UK) (2008) *Statement on Compression-Only Cardiopulmonary Resuscitation*. Resuscitation Council (UK), London.

Ruben H, Macnaughton F (1978) The treatment of food-choking. *Practitioner* **221**:725–9.

Ryan A, Larsen P, Galletly D (2003) Comparison of heart rate variability in supine, and left and right lateral positions. *Anaesthesia* **58**(5): 432–6.

Sans S, Kesteloot H, Kromhout D (1997) The burden of cardiovascular diseases mortality in Europe. Task Force of the European Society of Cardiology on Cardiovascular Mortality and Morbidity Statistics in Europe. *European Heart Journal* **18**:1231–48.

Sayre M, Berg R, Cave D *et al.* (2008) Hands-only (compression-only) CPR: a call to action for bystander response to adults who experience out-of-hospital sudden cardiac arrest. A science advisory for the public from the American Heart Association Emergency Cardiovascular Care Committee. *Circulation* published online 31 March 2008: http://circ.ahajournals.org/cgi/reprint/CIRCULATIONAHA.107.189380

Turner S, Turner I, Chapman D *et al.* (1997) A comparative study of the 1992 and 1997 recovery positions for use in the UK. *Resuscitation* **39**:153–60.

Wenzel V, Idris A, Banner M *et al.* (1994) The composition of gas given by mouth-to-mouth ventilation during CPR. *Chest* **106**:1806–10.

Yannopoulos D, McKnite S, Aufderheide T *et al.* (2005) Effects of incomplete chest wall decompression during cardiopulmonary resuscitation on coronary and cerebral perfusion pressures in a porcine model of cardiac arrest. *Resuscitation* **64**:363–72.

Yu T, Weil M, Tang W *et al.* (2002) Adverse outcomes of interrupted precordial compression during automated external defibrillation. *Circulation* **106**:368–72.

Chapter 6

Airway Management and Ventilation

Jagtar Singh Pooni and Phil Jevon

Introduction

Failure of the circulation for 3–4 minutes (less if the patient is initially hypoxaemic) can lead to irreversible cerebral damage. Restarting the heart following a cardiac arrest may not be possible without adequate reoxygenation (Resuscitation Council (UK), 2006).

Patients who require resuscitation often have airway obstruction, usually secondary to loss of consciousness, but sometimes it may be the primary cause of the cardiorespiratory arrest (Nolan *et al.*, 2005). Airway obstruction can be subtle and is often undetected by healthcare professionals (Nolan *et al.*, 2005).

Nurses must be competent at airway management and ventilation. Whatever the cause, prompt recognition and effective treatment of airway obstruction are essential, particularly during resuscitation, as an open and clear airway is essential to help ensure adequate ventilation.

The aim of this chapter is to understand the principles of airway management and ventilation.

Learning outcomes

At the end of the chapter the reader will be able to:

- List the causes of airway obstruction
- Outline the recognition of airway obstruction
- Describe simple techniques to open and clear the airway
- Discuss the procedure for the application of cricoid pressure

- Discuss the use of oropharyngeal and nasopharyngeal airways
- Outline the role of the laryngeal mask airway (LMA) and combitube
- Describe the procedure for endotracheal intubation
- Describe two methods of ventilation

Causes of airway obstruction

Causes of airway obstruction include:

- *Displaced tongue* – causes include unconsciousness, cardiac arrest and trauma
- *Fluid* – e.g. vomit, secretions and blood
- *Foreign body*
- *Laryngeal oedema* – causes include anaphylaxis and infection
- *Bronchospasm* – causes include asthma, foreign body and anaphylaxis
- *Trauma*
- *Pulmonary oedema* – causes include cardiac failure, anaphylaxis and near drowning

(Jevon, 2006)

Recognition of airway obstruction

Whatever the cause of airway obstruction, prompt recognition and effective management are essential. Recognition is best achieved by following the familiar look, listen and feel approach (Resuscitation Council (UK), 2006):

- *Look* for movements of the chest and abdomen
- *Listen* at the mouth and nose for airflow
- *Feel* at the mouth and nose for airflow

Airway obstruction can be partial or complete, and can occur at any level from the nose and mouth down to the trachea (Jevon, 2006).

Partial airway obstruction

Partial airway obstruction is usually characterised by noisy breathing:

- *Gurgling* – presence of fluid, e.g. secretions in the main airways
- *Snoring* – partial occlusion of the pharynx by the tongue
- *Inspiratory stridor* – upper airway obstruction (at or above the level of the larynx), e.g. foreign body, laryngeal oedema
- *Expiratory wheeze* – lower airway obstruction, e.g. asthma

Complete airway obstruction

Complete airway obstruction in a patient who is making respiratory efforts is characterised by paradoxical chest and abdominal movements ('see-saw' breathing) – when the patient tries to breathe in, the chest is drawn inwards and the abdomen expands; the opposite happens when the patient tries to breathe out (Resuscitation Council (UK), 2006). Accessory muscle use may also be evident, e.g. neck and shoulder muscles.

Simple techniques to open and clear the airway

Head tilt, chin lift and jaw thrust are three manoeuvres that can improve the patency of the airway, which has been obstructed by the tongue or other upper airway structures, e.g. soft palate or epiglottis (Nolan *et al.*, 2005). As regurgitation of gastric contents and vomiting commonly occurs during resuscitation, suction is regularly required and proficiency in applying it is essential (Jevon, 2006).

Head tilt/chin lift

The head tilt/chin lift manoeuvre (Figure 6.1) is considered the most effective method of opening the airway of an unconscious patient (Idris *et al.*, 1996). In basic life support (BLS) it can achieve airway patency in 91% of cases (Guildner, 1976). By stretching the anterior tissues of the neck, it displaces the tongue forward, away from the posterior pharyngeal wall, and lifts the epiglottis

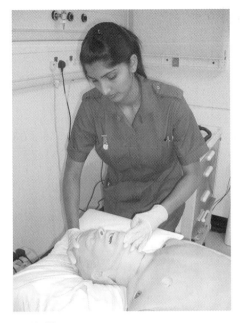

Fig. 6.1 Head tilt, chin lift.

from the laryngeal opening (Safar, 1958). A pillow under the head and shoulders can help to maintain this position.

To perform head tilt and chin lift:

1. Place one hand on the patient's forehead and gently tilt the head back
2. Place the fingertips of the other hand under the point of the patient's chin and lift the chin upwards

(Jevon, 2006)

Jaw thrust

The jaw thrust manoeuvre (Figure 6.2) is an alternative method to open the airway. It is recommended in patients with a suspected cervical spine injury, as head tilt may aggravate the injury

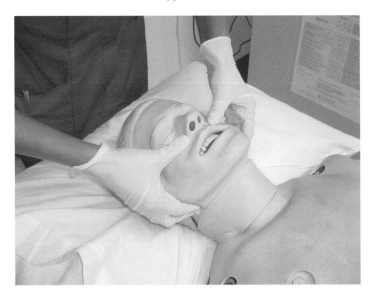

Fig. 6.2 Jaw thrust.

and damage the spinal cord (Donaldson *et al.*, 1997). When used in these patients, it should be accompanied by manual in-line immobilisation of the head and neck by an assistant (Nolan & Parr, 1997; Lennarson *et al.*, 2000). However, if life-threatening airway obstruction persists, despite the application of effective jaw thrust or chin lift, head tilt should be performed gradually more and more until airway patency is achieved: the establishment of a clear airway takes priority over concerns about potential injury to the cervical spine (Nolan *et al.*, 2005).

To perform a jaw thrust:

1. Using the index fingers positioned just proximal to the angles of the jaw, displace the mandible anteriorly (this will help to bring the tongue anteriorly)
2. Using the thumbs, apply pressure on the chin to help open the mouth

(Jevon, 2006)

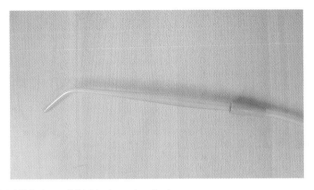

Fig. 6.3 Wide-bore rigid (Yankauer) catheter.

Suction

When obstruction is caused by vomit, secretions etc., simple BLS manoeuvres, such as placing the patient in the lateral position and finger sweeps, may help to clear the airway. A wide-bore rigid (Yankauer) catheter (Figure 6.3) can provide rapid suction of large volumes of fluid from the mouth and pharynx. A flexible catheter is particularly useful for suctioning down an oropharyngeal airway, nasopharyngeal airway and tracheal tube. In order to minimise deoxygenation, suction should last no longer than 10 seconds (Jevon, 2006).

A wall suction device is ideal for suction at the bedside (Figure 6.4). There are also several portable suction devices (Figure 6.5) currently available which are ideal in some situations, e.g. during patient transfer. Hand-held suction devices (Figure 6.6) can also be helpful.

Dentures

Well fitting dentures should be left in place because they will help to maintain the normal shape of the face, facilitating an adequate seal when ventilating using a bag/valve/mask device. However, displaced or broken dentures should be removed (Nolan *et al.*, 2005).

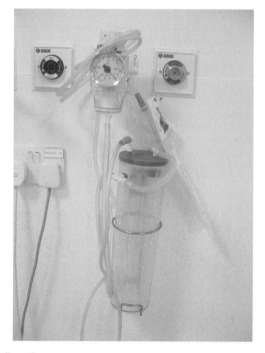

Fig. 6.4 Wall suction.

Use of oropharyngeal and nasopharyngeal airways

Oropharyngeal and nasopharyngeal airways are useful adjuncts because they can provide an artificial passage for airflow by separating the posterior pharyngeal wall from the tongue.

Oropharangeal airway

The oropharyngeal airway (Figure 6.7) can be used when there is obstruction of the upper airway due to the displacement of the tongue backwards and when glossopharyngeal and laryngeal reflexes are absent, e.g. during cardiopulmonary resuscitation (CPR).

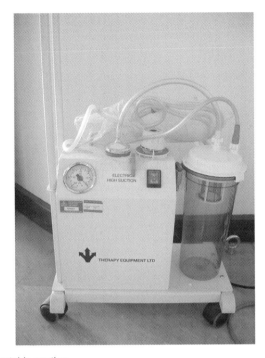

Fig. 6.5 Portable suction.

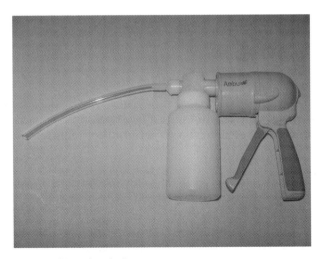

Fig. 6.6 Hand-held suction device.

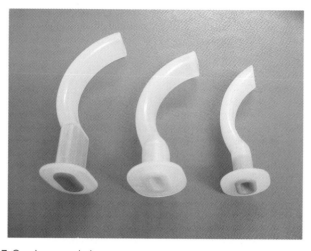

Fig. 6.7 Oropharangeal airways.

Cautions
- It should not be used in a patient who is not unconscious as it may induce vomiting and laryngospasm
- It should not be regarded as a definitive airway
- The correct size required should always be estimated
- The correct insertion technique should be adopted to minimise complications

Estimating the correct size
It is important to estimate the correct size. An oropharyngeal airway that is too big may occlude the airway by displacing the epiglottis, may hinder the use of a face mask and damage laryngeal structures; one that is too small may occlude the airway by pushing the tongue back.

An appropriate sized airway is one that holds the tongue in the normal anatomical position; following its natural curvature (Idris *et al.*, 1996). The curved body of the oropharyngeal airway is designed to fit over the back of the tongue.

The correct size is one that equates to the vertical distance from the angle of the jaw to the incisors (Nolan *et al.*, 2005); this can be estimated by placing the airway against the face and measuring

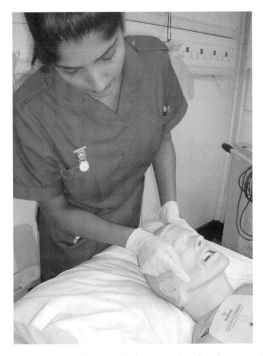

Fig. 6.8 Insertion of an oropharyngeal airway: estimating the correct size.

it from the patient's incisors to the angle of the jaw (Figure 6.8). A variety of different sizes are available, though normally sizes 2, 3 and 4 (Figure 6.7) are adequate for small, medium and large adults respectively (Resuscitation Council (UK), 2006).

Procedure for insertion
The correct insertion technique should be used in order to avoid unnecessary trauma to the delicate tissues in the mouth and inadvertently blocking the airway.

1. Don gloves (if available)
2. Clear the patient's airway, suction the mouth if necessary
3. Estimate the correct size by placing the airway against the patient's face and measuring it from the angle of the jaw to the incisors (Figure 6.8). The correct size required for the

patient is one that equates to the vertical distance between the incisors and the angle of the jaw (Nolan *et al.*, 2005). Oropharyngeal airway sizes 2, 3 and 4 are normally adequate for small, medium and large adults respectively (Nolan *et al.*, 2005)

4. If possible, lubricate the airway prior to insertion (practically, in the emergency situation, this is rarely done)
5. Open the patient's mouth, clear the airway, suction if necessary and insert the airway in the inverted position (Figure 6.9) (the curved part of the airway will help depress the tongue and prevent it from being pushed posteriorly)
6. As it passes over the soft palate, rotate the airway through 180 degrees (Figure 6.10)
7. Following insertion, confirm that the airway has been position correctly: the patient's airway should be improved and the flattened reinforced section should be positioned in between the patient's teeth, or gums if edentulous (Resuscitation Council (UK), 2006)
8. Closely monitor the patency and position of the airway; it can become blocked by the tongue or epiglottis and can become

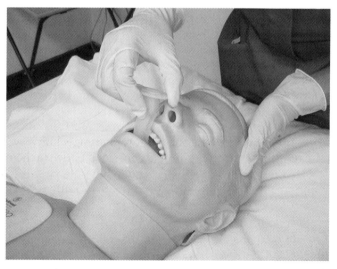

Fig. 6.9 Insertion of an oropharyngeal airway: open the patient's mouth, clear the airway suction if necessary and insert the airway in the inverted position.

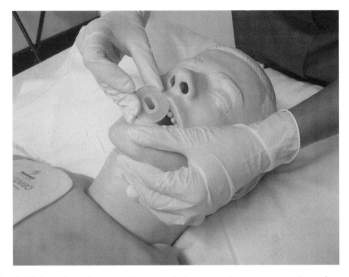

Fig. 6.10 Insertion of an oropharyngeal airway: as it passes over the soft palate, rotate the airway through 180 degrees.

wedged into the vallecula (Marsh *et al.*, 1991). Vomit, secretions and blood can also compromise its patency

(Jevon, 2006b)

Nasopharyngeal airway

The nasopharyngeal airway (Figure 6.11) is made from soft plastic with a flange at one end and a bevelled edge at the other. It is less likely to induce gagging than an oropharyngeal airway and it can be used in a semiconscious or conscious patient when the airway is at risk of being compromised (e.g. in the post-resuscitation period). It can be life saving in a patient with a clenched jaw, trismus or maxillofacial injuries (Jevon, 2006b).

Previously, the use of a nasopharyngeal airway has been contraindicated in patients with a suspected base of skull fracture, as it could penetrate the cranial fossa (Muzzi *et al.*, 1991). However, although an oropharyngeal airway is preferred in these patients, if it is not possible to insert it and the airway is obstructed, careful

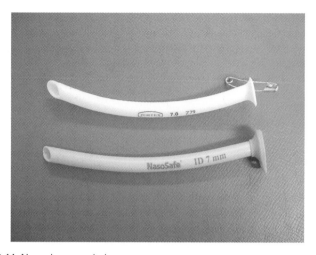

Fig. 6.11 Nasopharyngeal airway.

insertion of a nasopharyngeal airway could be life saving, i.e. the benefits may far outweigh the risks (Nolan *et al.*, 2005).

Insertion may damage the mucosal lining of the nasal airway, resulting in bleeding. The correct size should be used and prior to insertion, a safety pin should be securely inserted into the flange to prevent inhalation of the airway.

Estimating the correct size

It is important to estimate the correct size. If it is too short it will be ineffective and if it is too long it may enter the oesophagus, causing distension and hypoventilation or may stimulate the laryngeal or glossopharyngeal reflexes causing laryngospasm and vomiting (Jevon, 2006a).

The airways are sized in millimetres according to their internal diameter; the larger the diameter the longer the length. Traditionally, measurement against the patient's little finger or anterior nares were the recommended methods of determining which size nasopharyngeal airway to use (Nolan *et al.*, 2005). However, these methods are unreliable as they do not correlate well with the patient's airway anatomy (Roberts & Porter, 2003). In adults sizes 7–8 are used (Nolan *et al.*, 2005).

Procedure for insertion

1. Where appropriate explain the procedure to the patient
2. Select an appropriately sized airway
3. If necessary, insert a safety pin through the flange (some devices require this, a precautionary measure to prevent inhalation of the airway (Jevon, 2006a))
4. Check the right nostril for patency
5. Lubricate the airway
6. Insert the airway into the nostril, bevelled end first (Figure 6.12). Pass it vertically along the floor of the nose, using a slight twisting action, into the posterior pharynx. (If there is resistance remove the airway and try the left nostril.) Once inserted the flange which should be at the level of the nostril

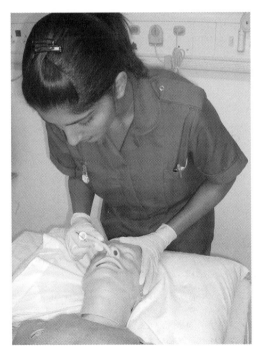

Fig. 6.12 Insertion of a nasopharyngeal airway: insert it into the nostril, bevelled end first.

7. Secure the airway with tape
8. Reassess the airway and check for patency and adequacy of ventilation. Continue to maintain correct alignment of the airway and chin lift as necessary and monitor the patency of the airway

(Jevon, 2006b)

Insertion of the laryngeal mask airway (LMA)

The LMA (Figure 6.13), which was first used in anaesthetic practice in the 1980s (Brain, 1983), is considered a first-line airway device during resuscitation, if expertise in tracheal intubation is not available (Resuscitation Council (UK), 2006). Successful ventilation following LMA insertion is reported to be 71–97% (American Heart Association, 2005). If the LMA can be inserted without delay, it is recommended to avoid bag--mask ventilation altogether (Nolan *et al.*, 2005).

The ProSeal LMA is a modification of the original LMA. It has a gastric drain and an additional posterior cuff, which, in theory, make it better and more effective than the standard LMA during

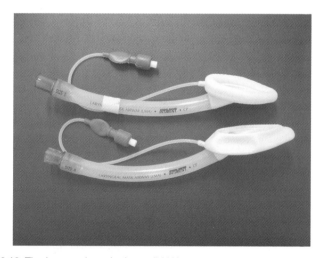

Fig. 6.13 The laryngeal mask airway (LMA).

CPR (Resuscitation Council (UK), 2006). Its use in CPR is being evaluated.

Description

The LMA is a curved, wide-bore tube with an inflatable cuff at the distal end, which is designed to seal around the laryngeal opening (Resuscitation Council (UK), 2006). Available in a variety of sizes, sizes 3, 4 and 5 are appropriate for small, average and large adults respectively (Resuscitation Council (UK), 2006). Single-use devices are usually used in resuscitation.

Advantages

Advantages of the LMA include:

- Enables securing the airway before tracheal intubation skills are available
- Can easily be taught to wide range of personnel, including nurses (American Heart Association, 2005)
- Ventilation using the LMA is more efficient and easier than with a bag–mask device (Alexander *et al.*, 1993)
- A simpler skill to learn and be proficient at than treacheal intubation because it does not require laryngoscopy and visualisation of the vocal cords (American Heart Association, 2005)
- Helpful in situations when tracheal intubation is difficult, e.g. when there is suspected cervical spine injury (restricted movement) (Pennant *et al.*, 1992), restricted access to the patient and inability to position patient appropriately (American Heart Association, 2005)

Airway protection

The LMA does not protect the airway from aspiration of gastric contents. However, gastric inflation (and subsequent regurgitation of gastric contents) is unlikely if high inflation pressures ($>20\,cmH_2O$) during ventilations are avoided (Resuscitation Council (UK), 2006). Regurgitation of gastric contents is less likely to occur with the LMA than with the bag–mask device and pulmonary aspiration is uncommon (American Heart Association, 2005).

Procedure for insertion

1. Move the bed away from the wall; remove the backrest to facilitate access (Resuscitation Council (UK), 2001)
2. Adopt a position at the top of the bed, facing the patent, with the feet in the walk/stand position (Resuscitation Council (UK), 2001). If it is not possible to approach the patient from the behind the head, the LMA can be inserted from the front (Resuscitation Council (UK), 2006)
3. Select an appropriately sized LMA: sizes 3, 4 and 5 are suitable for small, normal and large adults respectively
4. Completely deflate the cuff
5. Lubricate the outer cuff, i.e. the part that will not be in contact with the larynx
6. Ensure that the patient is in a supine position with the head and neck aligned
7. Extend the head and slightly flex the neck (unless cervical spine injury is suspected)
8. Holding the tube of the LMA like a pen, introduce the LMA into the mouth with the distal aperture facing towards patient's feet (Figure 6.14)
9. Using the index finger as a splint, advance the tip of the LMA, while applying its upper surface to the surface of the palate, until it reaches the wall of the posterior pharynx
10. While ensuring that the tube remains in the mid-line (the black line on the tube should be aligned with the patient's nasal septum), push the LMA backwards and downwards until it reaches the back of the pharynx and resistance is felt
11. Connect an appropriate syringe (usually 50 ml), let go of the LMA and inflate the cuff with the specified amount of air (20 ml, 30 ml and 40 ml for sizes 3, 4 and 5 respectively) If the LMA has been correctly inserted, the tube will lift out of the mouth slightly (1–2 cm) and the larynx is pushed anteriorly
12. Connect ventilatory device to the LMA, e.g. a self-inflating bag with oxygen supply
13. Confirm correct LMA placement by auscultating the chest during inflation and observe for bilateral chest movement (Figure 6.15). A small air leak is acceptable, though a large one would suggest malposition. If an adequate airway has not been achieved withdraw the LMA and start again, ensuring good insertion technique

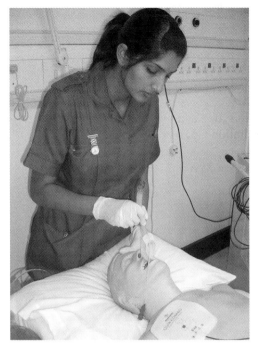

Fig. 6.14 Insertion of a LMA: holding the tube of the LMA like a pen, introduce the LMA into the mouth with the distal aperture facing towards patient's feet.

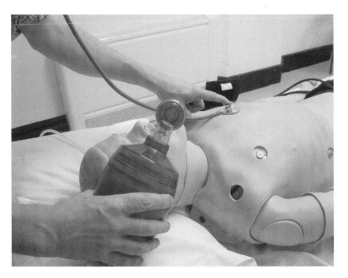

Fig. 6.15 Confirming correct placement of LMA: chest auscultation.

14. Insert a biteblock or oropharyngeal airway and secure the LMA with a 3 cm bandage.
15. While ventilating, adopt a comfortable position and avoid prolonged static postures (Resuscitation Council (UK), 2001)
16. Once the LMA is inserted, deliver continuous chest compressions without interruptions for ventilations (rate 10 per minute) (unless excessive air leakage results in ineffective ventilations, in which case revert to 30 chest compressions: two ventilations) (Nolan *et al.*, 2005)

(Nolan *et al.*, 2005; Jevon 2006c; Resuscitation Council (UK), 2006)

Complications

- Coughing, gagging, straining or laryngeal spasm can occur if the patient is not deeply unconscious
- Occasionally, during insertion of the LMA, the epiglottis can fold over the laryngeal inlet and occlude the airway
- Persistent air leakage can occur if the LMA is too small or if the cuff is not sufficiently inflated or if there is high airway resistance or poor lung compliance, e.g. pulmonary oedema, bronchospasm.

Insertion of the combitube

The combitube is a double-lumen tube, which is introduced blindly and designed to achieve ventilation whether it is placed into the trachea or oesophagus (Frass *et al.*, 1989). Following insertion, an assessment is then made of its position and the patient is then ventilated through the appropriate lumen. It has been used successfully as an airway adjunct in the cardiac arrest situation and has been used by paramedics in the pre-hospital situation (Atherton & Johnson, 1993).

Procedure for insertion

1. Position the patient in a supine position, with the head and neck in alignment

2. Open the patient's mouth and support the chin
3. Lubricate the combitube
4. Pass the combitube blindly over the tongue until the patient's teeth are between the two black ring markers on the tube
5. Inflate the large pharyngeal cuff with a maximum of 85 ml of air. The tube often moves up and down as the cuff is inflated
6. Inflate the distal cuff with 12 ml of air
7. Ventilate through the oesophageal channel (pilot balloon labelled No. 1) and look for any chest movement and abdominal distension and auscultate for breath sounds. If breath sounds are heard, continue ventilating through this channel
8. If breath sounds are not heard, ventilate through the tracheal channel (pilot balloon labelled No. 2). Auscultate for breath sounds

Procedure for application of cricoid pressure

Cricoid pressure helps to prevent the passive regurgitation and aspiration of gastric contents during bag–mask ventilation and attempted tracheal intubation (Nolan *et al.*, 2005). As well as being advocated during resuscitation, cricoid pressure is routinely used in other situations, e.g. emergency induction of general anaesthesia and prior to anaesthesia for caesarean section (Jevon, 2006a).

The application of cricoid pressure was first described in 1774, when it was used to prevent regurgitation and gastric distension during resuscitation of victims of drowning (Salem *et al.*, 1974). In the 1960s, Sellick provided the first in-depth description of the use of cricoid pressure in modern anaesthetic practice (Sellick, 1961). Sometimes cricoid pressure is referred to as 'the Sellick manoeuvre'.

Relevant anatomy

The cricoid cartilage, the first tracheal cartilage, is situated below the thyroid cartilage from which it is separated by the cricothyroid membrane (Bryant, 1999). It is the only complete ring of cartilage in the respiratory system (Koziol *et al.*, 2000). The other tracheal cartilages are C-shaped (i.e. incomplete rings of cartilage), which may collapse if pressure is applied (Feinstein & Owens, 1992).

Risk of regurgitation and pulmonary aspiration

During resuscitation, gastric inflation, together with an incompetent oesophageal sphincter, increase the risk of regurgitation and pulmonary aspiration (Nolan *et al.*, 2005).

The risk of regurgitation is higher in pregnancy, in obese patients and in patients with a 'full stomach', even those that have been fasted prior to surgery if there is delayed gastric emptying, e.g. bowel obstruction, trauma, opiate administration and trauma (Koziol *et al.*, 2000).

Impaired laryngeal function leading to diminished laryngeal sensation and protective airway reflexes will increase the risk of pulmonary aspiration.

Indications

Indications for cricoid pressure include:

- During CPR until the airway is secured by a cuffed tracheal tube
- Immediately prior to induction of general anaesthesia in the non-fasted patient
- Delayed gastric emptying
- Incompetent lower oesophageal sphincter, e.g. late pregnancy
- Difficult intubation – can help with the visualisation of the vocal cords

(Jevon, 2006a)

Amount of pressure

According to Mehrotra and Paust (1979), the appropriate amount of pressure applied to the cricoid is that which would cause pain if were to be applied to the bridge of the nose. Cheek and Gutsche (1993) suggest inability to swallow equates to appropriate cricoid pressure.

A more scientific approach can be used: cricoid pressure generates a force which can be expressed in newtons (N) (Koziol *et al.*, 2000); 9.81 N equates to the force of gravity on a mass of 1 kg (Parbrook *et al.*, 1990). For convenience, 10 N approximately equates to 1 kg (Vanner & Asai, 1999); 30 N (3 kg) of force needs to be applied to the cricoid in order to achieve oesophageal occlusion (Vanner & Pryle, 1992) (less when applied prior to induction).

Mode of action

When applied correctly, cricoid pressure compresses the proximal oesophageal lumen between the cricoid cartilage and the cervical vertebrae (Vanner, 1993), occluding the lumen of the oesophagus, helping to prevent regurgitation and aspiration of gastric contents. This will also minimise gastric inflation, which often occurs with bag–mask ventilation during CPR.

Procedure

1. Place a pillow under the patient's head and shoulders
2. Locate the cricoid cartilage – the first complete ring of cartilage below the thyroid cartilage (Adam's apple)
3. Using the dominant hand, place the index finger and thumb on either side of the cricoid cartilage (Figure 6.16)

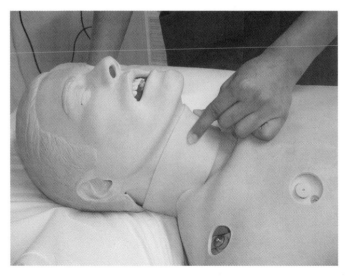

Fig. 6.16 Cricoid pressure: using the dominant hand, place the index finger and thumb on either side of the cricoid cartilage.

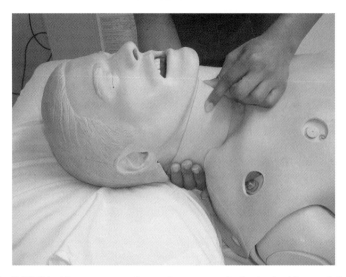

Fig. 6.17 Cricoid pressure: apply counter pressure to the back of the neck if there is a suspected cervical spine injury.

4. Apply cricoid pressure. Following pre-oxygenation, but prior to intravenous induction, apply a force of 10 N (1 kg) and, following loss of consciousness, increase the force to 30 N (3 kg) (this force should also be applied during CPR)
5. Apply counter pressure to the back of the neck if there is a suspected cervical spine injury (Figure 6.17). This will reduce movement of the cervical spine
6. Release cricoid pressure once a cuffed tracheal tube protects the airway, if the patient actively vomits or on the anaesthetist's request
7. If lung inflation is not possible, either reduce the pressure being applied or release the pressure completely (Nolan *et al.*, 2005)

Complications

Complications of cricoid pressure include:

• Retching and death from aspiration and ruptured oesophagus if excess force is applied in an awake patient

- Difficult tracheal intubation
- Difficult ventilation
- Aggravation of an existing cervical spine injury

(Heath *et al.*, 1996)

Cautions

Cricoid pressure should not be applied during active vomiting because there is a risk of damage to the oesophagus (Resuscitation Council (UK), 2006). When applied during tracheal intubation, too much pressure can distort the airway and may hinder the procedure.

Principles of tracheal intubation

During adult resuscitation, tracheal intubation is considered to be the optimum method of providing and maintaining a clear airway (Nolan *et al.*, 2005). The procedure, which can be difficult and sometimes hazardous, requires considerable skill and experience, particularly when performed in difficult circumstances, e.g. during CPR.

Advantages

Advantages of tracheal intubation include:

- Maintenance of a patent airway, which is protected from aspiration
- It is unnecessary to interrupt chest compressions while providing ventilations
- Provides an optional route for administration of certain resuscitation drugs, e.g. adrenaline, if intravascular access is delayed or not possible
- Ability to apply suction to the trachea and lower airways
- Enables the rescuer to undertake other tasks

(Nolan *et al.*, 2005).

Disadvantages

Disadvantages of tracheal intubation include:

- Difficult procedure to undertake; has a comparatively high failure rate (Nolan *et al.*, 2005)
- Unrecognised misplaced (or displaced) tracheal tube, e.g. into the oesophagus, will have disastrous consequences
- Interruption to chest compressions during the procedure

In some patients attempted tracheal intubation may actually lead to life-threatening deterioration, e.g. acute epiglottis pathology, cervical spine injury and head injury (straining could further increase intracranial pressure) (Nolan *et al.*, 2005). If the patient has a suspected cervical spine injury, it is important to maintain immobilisation of the cervical spine while performing tracheal intubation.

Equipment

A suggested list of equipment includes:

- Working laryngoscope with a curved Macintosh blade (size 3 is usually adequate); spares immediately available
- Cuffed tracheal tubes (normally a 7.0 for a woman and 8.0 for a man is sufficient)
- Suction source, together with both rigid and wide-bore (Yankauer), and flexible catheters
- Oxygen source
- Water-soluble lubricating jelly
- Introducer – either a gum elastic bougie or stylet
- Syringe to inflate the cuff on tracheal tube
- Tape or bandage to secure the tube
- Ventilatory device, e.g. bag–mask device
- Stethoscope
- Exhaled carbon dioxide device or oesophageal detector device (to confirm placement of tracheal tube)

(Resuscitation Council (UK), 2006)

Procedure

1. Move the bed away from the wall and remove the backrest
2. Assemble the necessary equipment and ensure good working order
3. Adopt a position at the top of the bed facing the patient with the feet in the walk/stand position (Resuscitation Council (UK), 2001)
4. Pre-oxygenate the patient with at least 85% oxygen for a minimum of 15 seconds
5. Ensure the patient is in the supine position with the neck slightly flexed and the head extended. A pillow under the head and shoulders can help to achieve this position
6. Ensuring the light source is on, hold the laryngoscope in the left hand and gently insert it into the righthand corner of the patient's mouth. Take care that the lower lip is not caught between the teeth and the blade
7. Advance the laryngoscope blade into the mouth, sweeping the tongue to the left in the process (Figure 6.18)

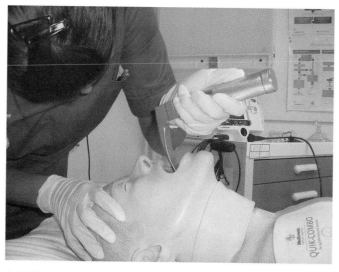

Fig. 6.18 Tracheal intubation: advance the laryngoscope blade into the mouth, sweeping the tongue to the left in the process.

8. Position the tip of the blade in the vallecula (area between the back of the tongue and the base of the epiglottis)
9. Lift upwards along the line of the laryngoscope handle. This should lift the epiglottis out of the way, revealing the vocal cords. Suction if necessary
10. Insert the tracheal tube (ideally lubricated) from the right-hand side of the mouth through the vocal cords (chest compressions will need to be briefly stopped), positioning the cuff just below the vocal cords (this usually equates to 21 cm and 23 cm marks on the tracheal tube in women and men respectively, measured at the patient's incisors) (Resuscitation Council (UK), 2006)
11. Inflate the tracheal tube cuff with sufficient air (usually 7–10 ml) to stop the audible leak associated with ventilation
12. Connect to a ventilatory device (often via a catheter mount) and ventilate with high-flow oxygen (Figure 6.19)
13. Confirm correct tube placement (see below). If air entry is only detected in the right side of the chest, this may indicate intubation of the right main bronchus: deflate the cuff, withdraw the tube 1–2 cm, reinflate cuff and reassess (Resuscitation Council (UK), 2006)

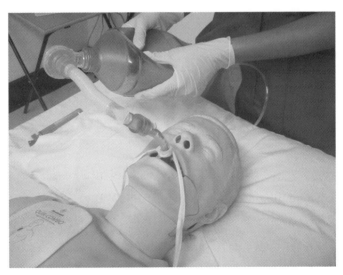

Fig. 6.19 Tracheal intubation: connect to a ventilatory device (often via a catheter mount) and ventilate with high-flow oxygen.

14. Secure the tube and continue ventilation and continually reassess tube position
15. Adopt a comfortable position and avoid prolonged static postures (Resuscitation Council (UK), 2001)
16. Ensure that the tracheal intubation attempt does not take longer than 30 seconds (Nolan *et al.*, 2005)

(Source: Jevon, 2006c)

Tracheal intubation in a patient collapsed on the floor

If undertaking tracheal intubation in a patient who has collapsed on the floor:

- Kneel behind the head of the patient, ensuring the knees are shoulder-width apart
- Bend forwards from the hips over the patient's head
- Resting the elbows on the floor may provide a more stable position

(Resuscitation Council (UK), 2001)

Confirmation of correct tracheal tube placement

Clinical signs of correct tracheal tube placement, e.g. tube condensation, chest rise, breath sounds on chest auscultation and inability to hear gas sounds entering the stomach, are not 100% reliable (Nolan *et al.*, 2005). In addition to the standard checks, the use of an exhaled carbon dioxide device or an oesophageal detector device will minimise the risk of undetected oesophageal intubation.

Ineffective ventilation following tracheal intubation

Effective ventilation may not be established following tracheal intubation or if it is may become ineffective after a variable period (Resuscitation Council (UK), 2006). The main causes of this can be described by the acronym DOPE:

- **D**isplaced tube. Either into pharynx/oesophagus, right/left main bronchus

- Obstructed tube. Vomit, blood, secretions and kinked tube
- Pneumothorax
- Equipment failure

(Jevon, 2002)

These problems should be recognised by the checks that routinely follow tracheal intubation.

Methods for ventilation

> Note: the most common cause of failure to ventilate is improper positioning of the head and chin (Idris *et al.*, 1996).

Although chest compressions are now given priority over ventilations during the initial resuscitation sequence (Kern *et al.*, 2002; Handley *et al.*, 2005), effective ventilations are still required and are indeed essential in prolonged arrests if cerebral function is to be maintained and the chance of survival is to be optimised.

Mouth-to-mouth ventilation

It is rarely necessary to have to perform mouth-to-mouth resuscitation, certainly in the hospital environment. At the very least a pocket mask should always be immediately available (Soar & Spearpoint, 2005).

Mouth-to-mouth ventilation has been described in Chapter 5. It must be stressed that although mouth-to-mouth ventilation is effective, it is only possible to deliver 16–17% oxygen to the patient; a ventilatory device with supplementary oxygen should be used as soon as practically possible.

Mouth-to-mask ventilation (pocket mask)

The pocket mask (Figure 6.20) is an excellent first-response device. It is transparent, thus enabling prompt detection of vomit or blood in the patient's airway. A one-way valve directs the patient's expired air away from the nurse.

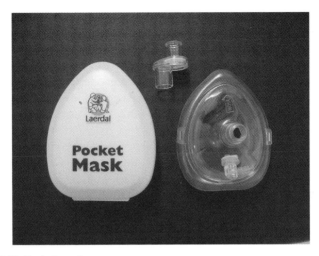

Fig. 6.20 Pocket mask.

Most pocket masks have an oxygen connector for the attachment of supplementary oxygen (10 l/min) (Resuscitation Council (UK), 2006), enabling an inspired oxygen concentration of approximately 50% being achieved. If there is no oxygen connector, supplementary oxygen can still be added by placing the oxygen tubing underneath one side of the mask and pressing down to achieve a seal (Nolan *et al.*, 2005).

Procedure for mouth-to-mask ventilation
1. Don gloves (if available)
2. Kneel behind the patient's head, ensuring the knees are shoulder-width apart (if alone kneel at the side of the patient level with his nose and mouth) (Resuscitation Council (UK), 2001)
3. Rest back to sit on the knees and adopt a low kneeling position (Resuscitation Council (UK), 2001)
4. Bend forwards from the hips, leaning down towards the patient's face and resting the elbows on your legs to support your weight (Resuscitation Council (UK), 2001)
5. If available, attach oxygen to the oxygen connector on the mask at a rate of 10 l/min (Resuscitation Council (UK), 2000). If there is no oxygen connector, place the oxygen tubing

underneath one side of the mask and press down to achieve a seal (Nolan *et al.*, 2005)

6. Apply the mask to the patient's face; press down with the thumbs and lift the chin into the mask by applying pressure behind the angles of the jaw

7. Take a breath in and ventilate the patient with sufficient air to cause visible chest rise (Figure 6.21). Each ventilation should last 1 second

8. If the patient is on a bed or trolley (its height should already have been adjusted so that the patient is level between the knee and mid-thigh of the nurse performing chest compressions): stand at the side facing the patient, level with his nose and mouth and bend forwards from the hips to minimise flexion of the spine; the nurse's weight can also be supported by resting the elbows on the bed and leaning the legs against the side of the bed frame (Resuscitation Council (UK), 2001). If another nurse is performing chest compressions adopt a position at the top of the bed facing the patient

9. Always adopt a comfortable position for ventilation and avoid static postures (Resuscitation Council (UK), 2001)

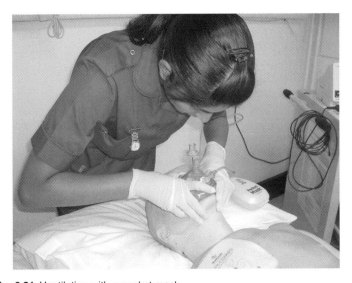

Fig. 6.21 Ventilation with a pocket mask.

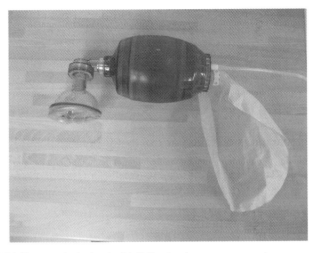

Fig. 6.22 Bag–mask device (self-inflating bag).

Bag–mask ventilation

The bag–mask (self-inflating bag) (Figure 6.22) device allows the delivery of higher concentrations of oxygen. If an oxygen reservoir bag is attached, with an oxygen flow rate of 10 l/min, an inspired oxygen concentration of approximately 85% can be achieved (Nolan *et al.*, 2005).

However, its use by a single person requires considerable skill. When used with a facemask, it can be difficult to achieve a seal with the mask, maintain an open airway and squeeze the bag (Alexander *et al.*, 1993). A two-person technique is therefore recommended, one person to open the airway and ensure a good seal with the mask, while the other squeezes the bag (Nolan *et al.*, 2005).

Procedure for bag–mask ventilation
1. Ensure the patient is supine.
2. Move the bed away from the wall and remove the backrest if applicable. Ensure the brakes of the bed are on. The height of the bed should be adjusted so that the patient is level between the knee and mid-thigh of the nurse performing chest compressions (Resuscitation Council (UK), 2001)

3. Adopt a position at the top of the bed facing the patient, with the feet in a walk/stand position (Resuscitation Council (UK), 2001)
4. Select an appropriately sized mask, i.e. it comfortably covers the mouth and nose, but does not cover the eyes or override the chin.
5. Ensure oxygen reservoir bag is attached and connect oxygen at a flow rate of 10 l/min (Nolan *et al.*, 2005)
6. First nurse: tilt the head back, apply the mask to the face, pressing down on it with the thumbs. Lift the chin into the mask by applying pressure behind the angles of the jaw. An open airway and an adequate face–mask seal should now be achieved. A pillow under the head and shoulders can help to maintain this position
7. Second nurse (positioned to the side of the bed): squeeze the bag (not the oxygen reservoir bag) sufficiently to cause visible chest rise (Figure 6.23). Each ventilation should be delivered over 1 second

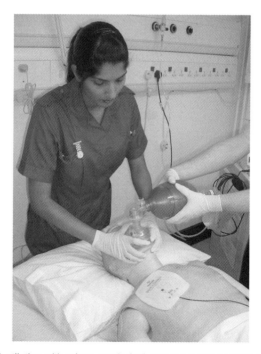

Fig. 6.23 Ventilation with a bag–mask device: two-person technique.

8. Observe for chest rise and fall. If the chest does not rise recheck the patency of the airway; slight readjustment may be all that is required
9. Adopt a comfortable position for ventilation and avoid static postures. Supporting your weight by resting your elbows on the bed may help (Resuscitation Council (UK), 2001)

Minimising gastric inflation

Excessive tidal volumes or inspiratory flows can generate excessive airway pressures, which can lead to gastric inflation and the subsequent risk of regurgitation and aspiration of gastric contents (Nolan *et al.*, 2005). It is therefore recommended to deliver each ventilation over 1 second, with sufficient volume to achieve chest rise, but avoiding rapid and forceful ventilations (Handley *et al.*, 2005).

Ineffective ventilations

If ventilations fail to achieve chest rise:

• Ensure adequate head tilt and chin lift
• Recheck the patient's mouth and remove any obstruction
• Ensure there is a good seal between the mask and the patient's face

Chapter summary

Effective airway management and ventilation are essential if oxygen supply to the brain is to be maintained during CPR. This chapter has described the principles of both basic and advanced techniques for airway management and ventilation.

References

Alexander R, Hodgson P, Lomax D, Bullen C (1993) A comparison of the laryngeal mask airway and guedel airway, bag and face mask for manual ventilation following formal training. *Anaesthesia* **48**:231–4.
American Heart Association (2005) Guidelines for cardiopulmonary resuscitation and emergency cardiovascular care. *Circulation* **112**(24) suppl:1–5.

Atherton G, Johnson JC (1993) Ability of paramedics to use the combi-tube in prehospital cardiac arrest. *Annals of Emergency Medicine* **22**:1263–8.

Brain A (1983) The laryngeal mask - a new concept in airway management. *British Journal of Anaesthesia* **55**:801–5.

Bryant A (1999) The use of cricoid pressure during emergency intubation. *Journal of Emergency Nursing* 25(4):283–4

Cheek T, Gutsche B (1993) Pulmonary aspiration of gastric contents. In: Shnider S, Levinson G (Eds) *Anesthesia for Obstetrics*, 3rd Ed. Williams & Wilkins, Baltimore.

Donaldson W, Heil B, Donaldson V, Silvaggio V (1997) The effect of airway maneuvers on the unstable C1-C2 segment. A cadaver study. *Spine* **22**:1215–8.

Feinstein R, Owens W (1992) Anesthesia for ear, nose and throat surgery. In: Barash P *et al.* (Eds) *Clinical Anesthesia*, 2nd Ed. Lippincott, Philadelphia.

Frass M, Frenzer R, Rauscha R et al (1989) Esophageal tracheal combi-tube, endotracheal airway and mask: comparison of ventilatory pressure curves. *Journal of Trauma* **29**:1476–9.

Guildner CW (1976) Resuscitation – opening the airway: a comparative study of techniques for opening an airway obstructed by the tongue. *Journal of the American College of Emergency Physicians* **5**:588–90.

Handley A, Kester R, Monsieurs K *et al* (2005) European Resuscitation Council Guidelines for Resuscitation 2005: Section 2. Adult basic life support and use of automated external defibrillators. *Resuscitation* **67S1**:S7-S23

Heath K, Palmer M, Fletcher S (1996) Fracture of cricoid cartilage after Sellick's manoeuvre. *British Journal of Anaesthesia* **76**:877–8.

Idris AH, Florete OG Jr, Melker RJ *et al.* (1996) Physiology of ventilation, oxygenation and carbon dioxide elimination during cardiac arrest. In: Paradis NA, Halperin HR, Nowak RM (Eds) *Cardiac Arrest: the Science and Practice of Resuscitation Medicine*. Williams & Wilkins, London.

Jevon P (2002) *Advanced Cardiac Life Support*, Butterworth Heinemann, Oxford.

Jevon P (2006) Resuscitation skills – part 2: clearing the airway. *Nursing Times* **102**(26):26–7.

Jevon P (2006a) Resuscitation skills – part 3: basic airway management. *Nursing Times* **102**(27):26–7.

Jevon P (2006b) Laryngeal mask airway. *Nursing Times* **102**(36):28–9.

Jevon P (2006c) Cricoid pressure. *Nursing Times* **102**(39):28–9.

Kern K, Hilwig R, Berg R *et al.* (2002) Importance of continuous chest compressions during cardiopulmonary resuscitation: improved outcome during a simulated single lay-rescuer scenario. *Circulation* **105**:645–9.

Koziol C, Cuddeford J, Moos D (2000) Assessing the force generated with application of cricoid pressure. *AORN Journal* **72**(6):1018–30.

Lennarson P, Smith D, Sawin P *et al.* (2000) Cervical spine motion during intubation: efficacy of stabilization maneuvers in the setting of complete segmental instability. *Journal of Neurosurgery. Spine* **94**:265–70.

Marsh A, Nunn J, Taylor S, Charlesworth C (1991) Airway obstruction associated with the use of the Guedel airway. *British Journal of Anaesthesia* **67**:517–23.

Mehrotra D, Paust J (1979) Antacids and cricoid pressure in preventing regurgitation of gastric contents. *Anesthesiology* **32**:553–5.

Muzzi D, Losasso T, Cucchiara R (1991) Complication from a nasopharyngeal airway in a patient with a basilar skull fracture. *Anesthesiology* **74**:366–8.

Nolan J, Deakin C, Soar J *et al.* (2005) European Resuscitation Council Guidelines for Resuscitation 2005: Section 4. Adult advanced life support. *Resuscitation* **675S**:S39-S86.

Nolan JP, Parr MJA (1997) Aspects of resuscitation in trauma. *British Journal of Anaesthesia* **79**:226–40.

Parbrook G, Davis P, Parbrook E (1990) *Basic Physics and Measurement in Anaesthesia*, 3rd Ed. Butterworth Heinemann, Oxford.

Pennant JH, Walker MB (1992) Comparison of the endotracheal tube and laryngeal mask in airway management by paramedical personnel. *Anesthesia & Analgesia* **74**:531–4.

Resuscitation Council (UK) (2001) *Guidance for Safer Handling During Resuscitation in Hospitals*. Resuscitation Council (UK), London.

Resuscitation Council (UK) (2006) *Advanced Life Support Provider Manual*, 5th Ed. Resuscitation Council (UK), London.

Roberts K, Porter K (2003) How do you size a nasopharyngeal airway. *Resuscitation* **56**:19–23.

Safar P (1958) Ventilatory efficiency of mouth to mouth respiration: airway obstruction during manual and mouth to mouth artificial ventilation. *Journal of the American Medical Association* **167**:335.

Salem M, Sellick B, Elam J (1974) The historical background of cricoid pressure in anesthesia and resuscitation. *Anesthesia and Analgesia* **53**:230–2.

Sellick B (1961) Cricoid pressure to control regurgitation of stomach contents during induction of anaesthesia. *Lancet* **2**:404–6.

Soar J, Spearpoint K (2005) In-hospital resuscitation. In: *Resuscitation Guidelines 2005*. Resuscitation Council (UK), London.

Vanner R (1993) Mechanisms of regurgitation and its prevention with cricoid pressure. *International Journal of Obstetric Anesthesia* **2**(4): 207–15

Vanner R, Asai T (1999) Safe use of cricoid pressure. *Anaesthesia* **54**:1–3.

Vanner R, Pryle B (1992) Regurgitation and oesophageal rupture with cricoid pressure: a cadaver study. *Anaesthesia* **47**:732–5.

Chapter 7

Defibrillation and Electrical Cardioversion

Introduction

The definitive treatment for a cardiac arrest caused by ventricular fibrillation (VF) or pulseless ventricular tachycardia (VT) is defibrillation. Defibrillation is the delivery of an electrical current across the myocardium of significant magnitude to depolarise a critical mass of the myocardium simultaneously to enable the restoration of organised electrical activity (Deakin & Nolan, 2005). A key component in the chain of survival (see Chapter 1), defibrillation is one of only two interventions that have been shown unequivocally to improve long-term survival following a cardiac arrest, the other being basic life support (BLS) (Resuscitation Council (UK), 2006).

Defibrillation has traditionally only been undertaken by doctors and senior nurses working in critical care areas. However the introduction of automated/advisory defibrillators has now made defibrillation possible by all nursing staff. All healthcare staff with a duty of care to perform cardiopulmonary resuscitation (CPR) should be trained, equipped and encouraged to perform defibrillation (and CPR) (Deakin & Nolan, 2005).

Synchronised electrical cardioversion is the delivery of a shock to the myocardium to terminate a tachyarrhythmia; to minimise the risk of inducing cardiac arrest the shock is timed (synchronised) so that it is delivered on the R wave and not during the vulnerable refractory period (T wave) (Jevon, 2006).

The aim of this chapter is to understand the principles of defibrillation and electrical cardioversion.

Learning objectives

At the end of this chapter the reader will be able to:

- Recognise ventricular fibrillation
- Discuss the physiology of defibrillation
- Outline the factors affecting successful defibrillation
- Discuss the safety issues related to defibrillation
- Describe the procedure for manual defibrillation
- Describe the procedure for automated external defibrillation
- Describe the procedure for synchronised electrical cardioversion
- Discuss the new technological advances in defibrillation

Ventricular fibrillation

The cardiac pump is thrown out of gear, and the last of its vital energy is dissipated in a violent and prolonged turmoil of fruitless activity in the ventricular walls.

(McWilliam, 1989)

In VF, the myocardium is depolarising at random resulting in uncoordinated electrical activity, with subsequent loss of cardiac output and cardiac arrest. Causes include myocardial ischaemia, electrolyte imbalance, hypothermia, drug toxicity and electric shock.

The electrocardiogram (ECG) trace is very characteristic with bizarre and chaotic waveforms. Initially coarse (Figure 7.1), the VF amplitude and waveform deteriorate rapidly reflecting the depletion of myocardial high energy phosphate stores (Mapin

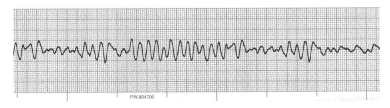

P/N 804700

Fig. 7.1 Ventricular fibrillation (coarse).

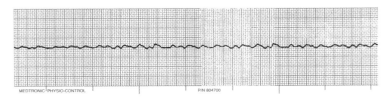

Fig. 7.2 Ventricular fibrillation (fine).

et al., 1991) with fine VF (Figure 7.2) and then asystole developing.

VF is the commonest primary arrhythmia at the onset of a cardiac arrest in adults (Resuscitation Council (UK), 2006). It is an eminently treatable rhythm with most eventual survivors of a cardiac arrest from this group (Resuscitation Council (UK), 2006). Early defibrillation is the definitive treatment; the chances of success decline substantially (7–10%) with each passing minute there is a delay to defibrillation (Waalewijn *et al.*, 2001). There is a slower decline if there is adequate BLS.

Physiology of defibrillation

The heart can respond to an extrinsic electrical impulse just as it can respond to an impulse from the sinoatrial (SA) node or from an ectopic focus. It is thought that successful defibrillation occurs when a critical mass of myocardium is depolarised by the passage of an electric current (Resuscitation Council (UK), 2006); if 75–90% of myocardial cells are in the repolarisation phase when the current is removed, successful defibrillation occurs and the SA node or another intrinsic pacemaker can then regain control.

Success will depend on the actual current flow rather than shock energy. This current flow is influenced by transthoracic impedance (resistance of the chest tissues), electrode position and shock energy delivered. Only a small proportion of the energy delivered actually reaches the myocardium; an effective defibrillation technique is essential to optimise the chances of successful defibrillation.

Factors affecting successful defibrillation

As well as early delivery following the onset of VF, there are several factors that can influence the likelihood of successful defibrillation. These will now be discussed.

Shock energy

Selecting the appropriate shock energy increases the likeliness of successful defibrillation, reduces the number of repetitive shocks and limits myocardial damage (Joglar *et al.*, 1999). Selecting the shock energy depends on whether the defibrillator is monophasic or biphasic:

- *Monophasic:* all shocks should be at 360 J
- *Biphasic:* 150–200 J for the first shock and 150–360 J for the second and all subsequent shocks – follow the manufacturer's recommendations and local policy

(Deakin & Nolan, 2005; Resuscitation Council (UK), 2006)

The three-shock sequence of shocks recommended in previous resuscitation guidelines has now been replaced by one shock; the rationale for this is the importance of minimising interruptions to CPR (Resuscitation Council (UK), 2006).

If a shockable rhythm (recurrent VF/pulseless VT) recurs, whether the interim ECG rhythm was associated with a cardiac output or not, the next shock energy to be selected should be the same one that had previously been successful (Deakin & Nolan, 2005).

Transthoracic impedance

If defibrillation is to be successful, sufficient electrical current needs to pass through the chest and depolarise a critical mass of myocardium. Transthoracic impedance is the resistance to the flow of current through the chest; the greater the resistance, the less the current flow. There are several factors that can influence transthoracic impedance and correct defibrillation technique is essential to minimise their effect and maximise current flow to the myocardium.

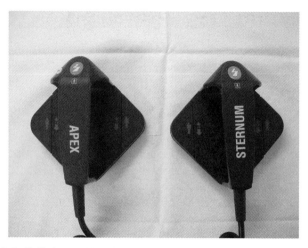

Fig. 7.3 Defibrillation paddle electrodes.

Electrode size: generally the larger the electrodes, the lower the impedance (Deakin *et al.*, 1999), though excessively large paddles can result in decreased current flow (Deakin *et al.*, 1999). The recommended sum of the electrode areas is a minimum of 150 cm² (Association of Instrumentation, 1993). In adult defibrillation, both handheld paddle electrodes (Figure 7.3) and self-adhesive pad electrodes (Figure 7.4) 8–12 cm in diameter are used and function well (Resuscitation Council (UK), 2006). Paediatric electrodes are associated with high impedance (Atkins & Kerber, 1992) and therefore should not be used in adults when larger paddles are available.

Shaving the chest: electrode-to-skin contact can be poor if the patient has a hairy chest as air can be trapped between the electrode and the skin; this can result in increased impedance, reduced defibrillation efficacy and arcing (sparks) causing burns to the patient's chest (Deakin & Nolan, 2005). If the patient has a hairy chest and a razor is immediately available, quickly remove hair from the area where the electrodes are going to be placed. N.B. if a razor is not immediately available, do not delay defibrillation (Resuscitation Council (UK), 2006).

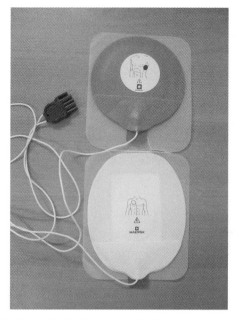

Fig. 7.4 Defibrillation self-adhesive pad electrodes.

Electrode paddles–skin interface: if electrode paddles are used with no electrode–skin interface, there will be high transthoracic impedance (Sirna *et al.*, 1988). Defibrillation gel pads (Figure 7.5) should be used to reduce the impedance between the electrode paddles and the skin (they also can help prevent skin burns). Defibrillation gel is not recommended because it can be messy and any 'stray' gel can lead to arcing on the chest and reducing the efficacy of defibrillation (Deakin & Nolan, 2005).

Electrode paddle force: if using electrode paddles, they should be pressed firmly to the chest wall as this will help to reduce impedance by improving electrical contact at the electrode–skin interface and reducing thoracic volume (Deakin *et al.*, 2002). In adults, the optimal electrode paddle force is 8 kg and, as this can be difficult to achieve, it is advisable for the strongest members of the cardiac arrest team to undertake this role (Deakin *et al.*, 2002).

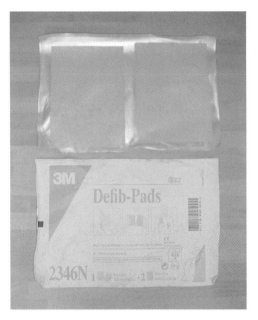

Fig. 7.5 Defibrillation gel pads.

Phase of ventilation: air is a poor conductor of electricity. There is reduced impedance when shocks are delivered at the end of full expiration compared to inspiration (Sirna *et al.*, 1988).

Electrode position: the electrodes should be placed to maximise the current flow through the myocardium. The polarity of the electrodes is unimportant for defibrillation (Bardy *et al.*, 1989; Deakin & Nolan, 2005), though for ECG monitoring and cardioversion they should be placed according to their namesakes (sternum and apex). If the apical electrode is oblong in shape, there will be reduced impedance if it is positioned longitudinally (Deakin *et al.*, 2003).

The most commonly used electrode position is one electrode on the anterior chest, just to the right of the sternum (not over the sternum) below the right clavicle, the other in the mid-axillary line approximately level with the V6 ECG electrode

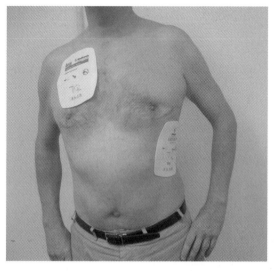

Fig. 7.6 Standard position for defibrillation electrodes placement.

position (Figure 7.6). In women, breast tissue should be avoided as this can increase transthoracic impedance (Pagan-Carlo *et al.*, 1996).

Other acceptable electrode positions include:

- *Anterior–posterior position:* (Figure 7.7) one electrode to the left of the lower sternal border and the other just below the left scapula. This technique can be difficult, particularly in a large patient. However it is advocated if defibrillation in the standard electrode position has been unsuccessful or if the patient has a permanent pacemaker or an implantable cardioverter defibrillator positioned below the right clavicle – the electrodes should be placed 12–15 cm away (Resuscitation Council (UK), 2006)
- *Bi-axillary position:* one electrode on each lateral chest wall (Deakin & Nolan, 2005)

The accuracy of electrode placement has been questioned and care should be taken to ensure correct placement.

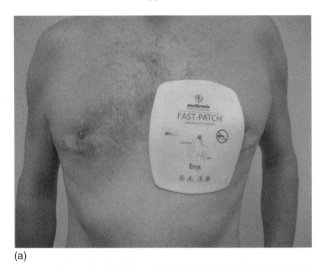

(a)

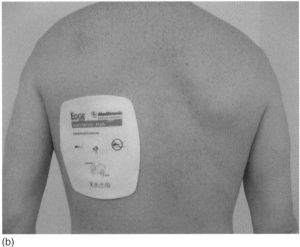

(b)

Fig. 7.7 Anterior (a) and posterior (b) position for defibrillation electrodes

Safety issues and defibrillation

General safety issues

- Confirm cardiac arrest and ascertain that the ECG trace displays a shockable rhythm

- Remove transdermal medication patches because they can compromise effective electrode contact and could cause arcing and burns (Wrenn, 1990)
- Avoid direct and indirect contact with the patient. All personnel should be well away from the bed and not touching the patient or anything attached to the patient/bed, e.g. intravenous infusion stands, intravenous infusions. Be wary of wet surroundings
- Temporarily remove oxygen delivery device at least 1 m away from the patient's chest (if the patient has a self-inflating bag connected to a tracheal tube or other airway device either leave it connected or remove it at least 1 m away form the patient's chest) (Resuscitation Council (UK), 2006). If the patient is on a ventilator, leave the ventilator tubing connected (Deakin & Nolan, 2005)
- Shout 'Stand clear' and check all personnel are safely clear prior to defibrillation. No person should be touching the patient or anything in contact with the patient, e.g. bed, drip stand
- Check the ECG monitor immediately prior to defibrillation; sometimes the ECG can revert to a non-shockable rhythm
- Place the defibrillation paddles 12–15 cm away from an implanted pacing unit (Resuscitation Council (UK), 2006) (most units are below the left clavicle, therefore the standard defibrillation can be adopted; if it is below the right clavicle the anterior–posterior paddle position may be necessary)
- Minimise the risk of sparks during defibrillation: in theory there is a decreased risk of this when using self-adhesive pad electrodes compared to paddle electrodes (Deakin & Nolan, 2005)

Safety issues when using adhesive electrode pads

- Ensure they are in date
- Ensure that the patient's chest is wiped dry
- Shave the chest if necessary (see above)

Safety issues when using electrode paddles

- Apply defibrillation gel pads to the patient's bare chest to minimise the risk of skin burns (and improve conduction)

- Apply adequate pressure to the paddles (8 kg) to help minimise the risk of arcing (Deakin *et al.*, 2002)
- Charge the defibrillator with the electrode paddles either on the patient's chest (preferable) or in their allocated storage site on the defibrillator
- If indicated, ask a colleague to increase the energy level on the defibrillator (if alone, return one electrode paddle to the defibrillator and use the free hand to increase the energy level)

Pads or paddles

Self-adhesive pad electrodes are safe, effective and preferable to paddle electrodes (Stults *et al.*, 1987). In addition, transthoracic impedance and efficacy are similar between the two systems (Kerber *et al.*, 1985). However, in hospital, pad electrodes are now becoming more commonplace as they have several distinct advantages including:

- Automated/advisory/manual defibrillation using the same system, i.e. first responder can use the defibrillator in the automated/advisory mode and the cardiac arrest team can then use the manual mode (depending on the defibrillator)
- Useful in clinical situations when access to the patient's chest is difficult (Deakin & Nolan, 2005)
- Enables the operator to defibrillate the patient 'hands-free' at a distance (electrode paddles require the operator to lean over the patient which is hazardous)
- Quicker than electrode paddles to establish ECG monitoring (Perkins *et al.*, 2002), i.e. ECG recognition and subsequent defibrillation will be performed quicker
- Not shown to be associated with spurious asystole, a problem encountered with electrode paddles when used for ECG monitoring following defibrillation (Chamberlain, 2000)

Procedure for manual defibrillation

Manual defibrillation using adhesive pad electrodes

The following procedure for manual defibrillation using adhesive pad electrodes is based on Resuscitation Council (UK) (2006) recommendations:

1. Confirm cardiac arrest and ensure the cardiac arrest team is alerted
2. Commence CPR, 30 compressions: two ventilations
3. As soon as the defibrillator arrives, switch it on and apply self-adhesive pad electrodes to the patient's bare chest following the manufacturer's recommendations – dry the chest, shave the electrode position site if necessary. The standard position for the electrodes is one on the anterior chest, just to the right of the sternum (not over the sternum) below the right clavicle, the other in the mid-axillary line approximately level with the V6 ECG electrode position (Figure 7.4)
4. Request that CPR is stopped and ascertain that the ECG rhythm is a shockable rhythm, i.e. VF/VT.
5. Select the correct energy level, i.e. 150–200 J biphasic (360 J monophasic) for the first shock and 150–360 J biphasic (360 J monophasic) for subsequent shocks following manufacturer's recommendations. Some defibrillators, when switched on, will default to the appropriate energy level
6. Press the charge button on the defibrillator and shout 'Stand clear'
7. Perform a visual check of the area to ensure that all personnel are clear
8. Check the monitor to ensure that the patient is still in VF/VT
9. Press both discharge button(s) simultaneously to discharge the shock (Figure 7.8)
10. Recommence CPR, 30 compressions: two ventilations
11. After 2 minutes, request that CPR is stopped and ascertain whether defibrillation is required; follow the Resuscitation Council (UK) advanced life support (ALS) algorithm (see Chapter 8, Figure 8.1)

Manual defibrillation using paddle electrodes

The following procedure for manual defibrillation using paddle electrodes is based on Resuscitation Council (UK) (2006) recommendations:

1. Confirm cardiac arrest and ensure the cardiac arrest team is alerted
2. Commence CPR, 30 compressions: two ventilations

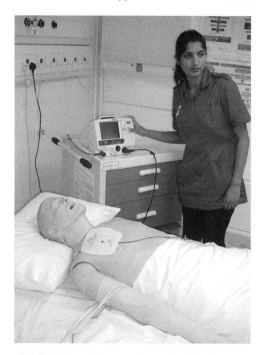

Fig. 7.8 Manual defibrillation using adhesive pad electrodes.

3. As soon as the defibrillator arrives, switch it on and apply defibrillation gel pads to the patient's bare chest (one on the anterior chest, just to the right of the sternum below the right clavicle, the other in the mid-axillary line approximately level with the V6 ECG electrode position) and apply paddle electrodes (Figure 7.3)
4. Request that CPR is stopped and ascertain that the ECG rhythm is a shockable rhythm, i.e. VF/VT
5. Select the correct energy level, i.e. 150–200J biphasic (360J monophasic) for the first shock and 150–360J biphasic (360J monophasic) for subsequent shocks following manufacturer's recommendations. Some defibrillators, when switched on, will default to the appropriate energy level
6. Press the charge button on the paddle electrodes and shout 'Stand clear'

7. Check all personnel are safely clear prior to defibrillation. No person should be touching the patient or anything in contact with the patient, e.g. bed, drip stand
8. Perform a visual check of the area to ensure that all personnel are clear
9. Once the defibrillator is charged, check the monitor to ensure that the patient is still in VF/VT
10. Press both discharge button(s) simultaneously to discharge the shock (Figure 7.9)
11. Return paddle electrodes to the defibrillator, ensuring CPR 30 compressions: two ventilations is immediately recommenced for 2 minutes
12. When monitoring the ECG through paddle electrodes, spurious asystole may be seen following the delivery of a shock (Resuscitation Council (UK), 2006), therefore attach ECG leads and select lead II as soon as possible

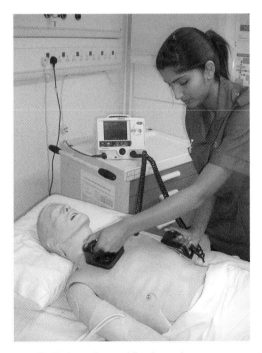

Fig. 7.9 Manual defibrillation using paddle electrodes.

13. After 2 minutes, request that CPR is stopped and ascertain whether defibrillation is required; follow the Resuscitation Council (UK) ALS algorithm (2006) (see Figure 8.1)

Procedure for automated external defibrillation

Operating a manual defibrillator requires extensive training and knowledge. Its use has therefore been traditionally restricted to doctors, and senior nurses working in critical care areas. However modern automated external defibrillators (AEDs) abolish the need for the operator to have ECG interpretation skills and spoken and/or visual prompts are provided.

As less operator training is required compared to manual defibrillators, they can be used by a wider range of personnel. More and more hospitals are now introducing this new technology to general wards, clinics etc. Early defibrillation by ward staff, before the arrival of the cardiac arrest team, should now be commonplace.

The following procedure for automated external defibrillation is based on Resuscitation Council (UK) (2006) recommendations:

1. Confirm cardiac arrest and ensure the cardiac arrest team (or similar) is alerted
2. Switch on AED and follow spoken and/or visual prompts
3. Prepare the patient's skin as necessary; ensure that the skin is dry and quickly remove any excess chest hair. If the patient has a hairy chest, the defibrillation electrodes may stick to the hairs resulting in high transthoracic impedance (Bissing & Kerber, 2000)
4. Apply self-adhesive pad electrodes to the patient's bare chest following the manufacturer's recommendations; the standard position for the position of the electrodes is one on the anterior chest, just to the right of the sternum (not over the sternum) below the right clavicle, the other in the mid-axillary line approximately level with the V6 ECG electrode position (Figure 7.4)
5. Stop CPR and ensure nobody is touching the patient during ECG analysis by the AED. This is to prevent artefactual errors during ECG analysis (Resuscitation Council (UK), 2006). Some

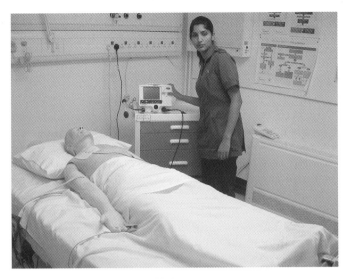

Fig. 7.10 Automated external defibrillation.

AEDs require the operator to press an 'analyse' button, while others automatically begin analysis once the self-adhesive pad electrodes are attached to the patient's chest

6. If shock is advised shout 'Stand clear' and perform visual check to ensure all staff are clear
7. Check all personnel are safely clear prior to defibrillation. No person should be touching the patient or anything in contact with the patient, e.g. bed, drip stand
8. Press shock button as indicated (if the AED is fully automated, it will deliver the shock automatically) (Figure 7.10)
9. Continue CPR 30 compressions: two ventilations as guided by the voice/visual prompts

Shock advisory defibrillators

Shock advisory defibrillators have ECG-analysis capability, but can be manually over-ridden by healthcare practitioners trained in ECG interpretation, e.g. members of the cardiac arrest team (Resuscitation Council (UK), 2006). Defibrillators with this facility are common in the hospital environment because they enable early defibrillation by the first responder (advisory facility) and then, when they arrive, defibrillation by the cardiac arrest team (manual facility), without having to change defibrillators.

Synchronised electrical cardioversion

Synchronised electrical cardioversion (SEC) is a reliable method of converting a tachyarrhythmia to sinus rhythm (Resuscitation Council (UK), 2006). Due to the associated risks, it is generally only undertaken when pharmacological intervention has been unsuccessful or if there are adverse signs, e.g. chest pain, hypotension, reduced level of consciousness, rapid ventricular rate and dyspnoea.

SEC is the delivery of a shock to the myocardium to terminate a tachyarrhythmia. To minimise the risk of inducing cardiac arrest the shock is timed (synchronised) so that it is delivered on the R wave.

Indications

SEC is indicated if the patient has a tachyarrhythmia and is unstable and compromised, for example with impaired consciousness, chest pain, heart failure, hypotension or other signs of shock (Nolan *et al.*, 2005). It can also be considered if drug therapy is ineffective.

Synchronisation with the R wave

The shock must be delivered with the R wave and not the T wave (Deakin & Nolan, 2005), as delivery of the shock during the refractory period of the cardiac cycle (T wave) could induce VF (Lown, 1967). The defibrillator must therefore be synchronised with the patient's ECG.

Sometimes synchronisation can be difficult in VT. If the patient is unstable the shock should be delivered unsynchronised to avoid a prolonged delay in restoring sinus rhythm (Resuscitation Council (UK), 2006).

Monophasic and biphasic waveforms

For cardioversion of a broad complex tachycardia and atrial fibrillation, 120–150 J biphasic (200 J monophasic) is recommended initially. For cardioversion of a regular narrow complex tachycardia or atrial flutter, lower energy levels are usually successful (70–120 J biphasic and 100 J monophasic are recommended initially) (Resuscitation Council (UK), 2005).

Safety considerations

Due to the risk of a cerebral embolism arising from stasis of blood in the left atrium, a patient who has had atrial fibrillation for more than 48 hours should normally not receive SEC until she or he has been fully anti-coagulated, or if transoesophageal echocardiography has confirmed the absence of an atrial clot (Resuscitation Council (UK), 2006).

Procedure

1. Record a 12-lead ECG, unless the patient is severely compromised and doing so will delay the procedure
2. Explain the procedure to the patient. Consent should be obtained if possible. If the patient is not unconscious, he must be anaesthetised or sedated for the procedure (Nolan *et al.*, 2005)
3. If necessary, shave the patient's chest (see above) as this can reduce transthoracic impedance (Sado *et al.*, 2004)
4. Ensure the resuscitation equipment is immediately available
5. Establish ECG monitoring using the defibrillator that will be used for cardioversion
6. Select an ECG monitoring lead that will provide a clear ECG trace, e.g. lead II.
7. Press the 'synch' button on the defibrillator
8. Check the ECG trace to ensure that only the R waves are being synchronised (Figure 7.11), i.e. a 'synchronised' dot or arrow should appear on each R wave and nowhere else on the PQRST cycle, e.g. on tall T waves
9. Apply defibrillation gel pads to the patient's chest, one just to the right of the sternum, below the right clavicle, and the other in the mid-axillary line, approximately level with the V6 ECG electrode or female breast (Deakin & Nolan, 2005)
10. Select the appropriate energy level on the defibrillator (see above for recommended levels)

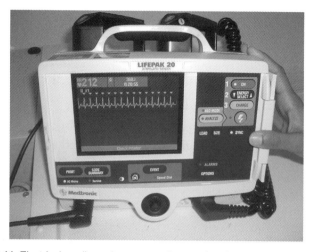

Fig. 7.11 Electrical cardioversion: ensure the synchronised button is activated.

11. Position the defibrillator paddles firmly on the defibrillation pads
12. Charge the defibrillator and shout 'Stand clear'
13. Check all personnel are safely clear prior to defibrillation. No person should be touching the patient or anything in contact with the patient, e.g. bed, drip stand
14. Check the ECG monitor to ensure that the patient is still in the tachyarrhythmia that requires cardioversion, that the synchronised button remains activated and that it is still synchronising with the R waves
15. Press both discharge buttons simultaneously to discharge the shock. There is usually a slight delay between pressing the shock buttons and shock discharge
16. Reassess the ECG trace. The 'synch' button will usually need to be reactivated if further cardioversion is required (on some defibrillators it is necessary to actually switch off the 'synch' button if further cardioversion is not indicated). Stepwise increases in energy will be required if cardioversion needs to be repeated (Deakin & Nolan, 2005). Amiodarone is indicated if three attempts at cardioversion have been unsuccessful (Nolan *et al.*, 2005)
17. After successful cardioversion, record a 12-lead ECG

18. Monitor the patient's vital signs until they have fully recovered from the anaesthetic or sedative

New technological advances in defibrillation

Implantable cardioverter defibrillator

The implantable cardioverter defibrillator (ICD) (Figure 7.12) can be used in patients with recurrent life-threatening ventricular arrhythmias who have not responded to conventional treatment. Its use is associated with improved chances of survival (Resuscitation Council (UK), 2006).

The ICD is positioned in a similar position to permanent pacemakers and can provide over-ride pacing, low-energy synchronised cardioversion, high-energy defibrillation and pacing for bradycardia (Causer & Connelly, 1998).

If a patient with an ICD has a cardiac arrest, standard CPR can be carried out without any risks to the team. If the ICD discharges it will not be detected by those carrying out the CPR. If external defibrillation is indicated, the paddles should be placed 12–15 cm away from the unit (Resuscitation Council (UK), 2006).

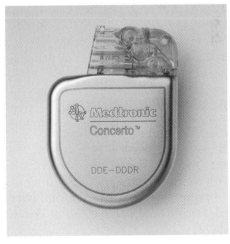

Fig. 7.12 Implantable cardioverter defibrillator (ICD). Reproduced with kind permission of Medtronic Ltd, Watford, UK (www.medtronic.com).

Biphasic waveform defibrillation

Older defibrillators have a monophasic waveform, i.e. the shock travels from one paddle electrode to the other. Newer defibrillators have a biphasic waveform, i.e. the shock travels from one electrode paddle to the other and then back again (Page *et al.*, 2002).

In defibrillation by ICDs, biphasic waveforms have been shown to be superior to monophasic ones (Cummins *et al.*, 1998). Repeated lower-energy biphasic waveform shocks (200 J or less) have the same or indeed higher success rates for terminating VF than monophasic waveform shocks of increasing joulage (200, 300, 360 J) (Poole *et al.*, 1997). However the optimum energy levels for biphasic waveform defibrillation have yet to be determined.

There are obvious advantages of biphasic waveform defibrillation which are associated with lower shock energy levels:

- Less myocardial damage
- Potential safety hazards will be reduced
- Defibrillators can be smaller, lighter and more portable

However whether the short-term outcomes improve long-term survival has yet to be determined (Resuscitation Council (UK), 2006).

Chapter summary

Early defibrillation is a key component in the chain of survival. It has been shown unequivocally to improve long-term survival following a cardiac arrest. It should be delivered promptly, safely and effectively. The principles of defibrillation and synchronised electrical cardioversion have been discussed in this chapter.

References

Association of Instrumentation (1993) *American National Standard: Automatic External Defibrillators and Remote Controlled Defibrillators (DF39)*. Association of Instrumentation, Virginia.

Atkins DL, Kerber RL (1992) Pediatric defibrillation: current flow is improved by using adult paddle electrodes. *Circulation* **86**(suppl 1): 1235.

Bardy GH, Ivey TD, Allen MD (1989) Evaluation of electrode polarity on defibrillation efficacy. *American Journal of Cardiology* **63**:433–7.

Bissing J, Kerber R (2000) Effect of shaving the chest of hirsute subjects on transthoracic impedance to self-adhesive defibrillation electrode pads. *American Journal of Cardiology* **86**:587–9.

Causer J, Connelly D (1998) Implantable defibrillators for life-threatening ventricular arrhythmias. *British Medical Journal* **317**:762–3.

Chamberlain D (2000) Gel pas should not be used for monitoring ECG after defibrillation. *Resuscitation* **43**:159–60.

Cummins R, Hazinski M, Kerber R *et al.* (1998) Low-energy biphasic waveform defibrillation: evidence-based review applied to emergency cardiovascular care guidelines: a statement for healthcare professionals from the American Heart Association Committee on Emergency Cardiovascular Care and the Subcommittees on Basic Life Support, Advanced Life Support and Paediatric Life Support. *Circulation* **97**:1654–67.

Deakin C, McLaren R, Petley G *et al.* (1999) A comparison of transthoracic impedance using standard defibrillation paddles and self-adhesive defibrillation pads. *Resuscitation* **39**:43–6.

Deakin C, Sado D, Petley G, Clewlow F (2002) determining the optimal paddle force for external defibrillation. *American Journal of Cardiology* **90**:812–3.

Deakin C, Sado D, Petley G, Clewlow F (2003) Is the orientation of the apical defibrillation paddle of importance during manual external defibrillation? *Resuscitation* **56**:15–8.

Deakin C, Nolan J (2005) European Resuscitation Council Guidelines for Resuscitation 2005: Section 3. Electrical therapies: automated external defibrillators, defibrillation, cardioversion and pacing. *Resuscitation* **675S**:S25–S37.

Jevon P (2006) Resuscitation skills – part 6: synchronised electrical cardioversion. *Nursing Times* **102**(30):28–9.

Joglar J, Kessler D, Welch P *et al.* (1999) Effects of repeated electrical defibrillations on cardiac troponin I levels. *American Journal of Cardiology* **83**:270–2.

Kerber R, Martins J, Ferguson D *et al.* (1985) Experimental evaluation and initial clinical application of new self-adhesive defibrillation electrodes. *International Journal of Cardiology* **8**:57–66.

Lown B (1967) Electrical reversion of cardiac arrhythmias. *British Heart Journal* **29**:469–89.

Mapin D, Brown C, Dzuonczyk R (1991) Frequency analysis of the human and swine electrocardiogram during ventricular fibrillation. *Resuscitation* **22**:85–91.

McWilliam J (1989) Cardiac failure and sudden death. *British Medical Journal* **5**: 6–8.

Nolan J, Deakin C, Soar J *et al.* (2005) European Resuscitation Council guidelines for resuscitation 2005: Section 4. Adult advanced life support. *Resuscitation* **675S**:S39–S86.

Pagan-Carlo LA, Spencer KT, Robertson CE *et al.* (1996) Transthoracic defibrillation: importance of avoiding electrode placement directly on the female breast. *Journal of the American College of Cardiology* **27**:449–52.

Page R, Kerber RE, Russell JK *et al.* (2002) Biphasic versus monophasic shock waveform for cardioversion of atrial fibrillation: the results of an international randomised, double-blind multi-center trial. *Journal of the American College of Cardiology* **39**:1956–63.

Perkins G, Roberts C, Gao F (2002) Delays in defibrillation: influence of different monitoring techniques. *British Journal of Anaesthesia* **89**:405–8.

Poole J, White D, Kanz K *et al.* (1997) Low-energy impedance-compensating biphasic waveforms terminate ventricular fibrillation at high rates in victims of out-of-hospital cardiac arrest. *Journal of Cardiovascular Electrophysiology* **8**:1373–85.

Resuscitation Council (UK) (2005) *Resuscitation Guidelines 2005.* Resuscitation Council (UK), London.

Resuscitation Council (UK) (2006) *Advanced Life Support*, 5th Ed. Resuscitation Council (UK), London.

Sado D, Deakin C, Petley G, Clewlow F (2004) Comparison of the effects of removal of chest hair with not doing so before external defibrillation on transthoracic impedance. *American Journal of Cardiology* **93**:98–100.

Sirna SJ, Ferguson DW, Charbonnier F *et al.* (1988) Factors affecting transthoracic impedance during electrical cardioversion. *American Journal of Cardiology* **62**:1048–52.

Stults K, Brown D, Cooley F, Kerber R (1987) Self-adhesive monitor/defibrillation pads improve prehospital defibrillation success. *Annals of Emergency Medicine* **16**:872–7.

Waalewijn R, de Vos R, Tijssen J, Koster R (2001) Survival models for out-of-hospital cardiopulmonary resuscitation from the perspectives of the bystander, the first responder and the paramedic. *Resuscitation* **51**:113–22.

Wrenn K (1990) The hazards of defibrillation through nitroglycerin patches. *American Journal of Emergency Medicine* **19**:1327–8.

Chapter 8

Advanced Life Support

Introduction

Advanced life support (ALS) is the term used to describe the more specialised techniques employed to support breathing and circulation during cardiopulmonary resuscitation (CPR), as well as specific treatment used to try to restore cardiac output. Effective CPR and early defibrillation are the only two interventions that have been shown to improve survival following a cardiac arrest: attention must therefore be focused on these while undertaking ALS (Nolan *et al.*, 2005).

All nurses involved with in-hospital CPR should understand the Resuscitation Council (UK) ALS algorithm (Figure 8.1), whether they are just performing basic CPR and using an automated defibrillator or whether they are responsible for providing ALS. The ALS algorithm is universally applicable, though specific modifications are required to maximise the likelihood of success in some special situations (see Chapters 9 and 10).

The aim of this chapter is to understand the principles of ALS.

Learning objectives

At the end of the chapter the reader will be able to:

- Discuss the background to the Resuscitation Council (UK) ALS algorithm
- Discuss the treatment of potential reversible causes of cardiac arrest
- Describe two drug delivery routes during CPR
- Discuss the use of resuscitation drugs
- Outline the principles of external pacing

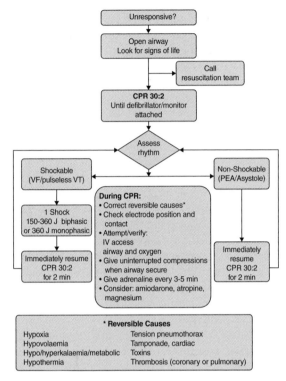

Fig. 8.1 Adult advanced life support algorithm. Reproduced with permission of Resuscitation Council (UK).

Background to the Resuscitation Council (UK) ALS algorithm

Ventricular fibrillation (VF)/pulseless ventricular tachycardia (VT) is the commonest primary arrhythmia at the onset of an adult cardiac arrest outside hospital (Resuscitation Council (UK), 2006). In hospital it is the presenting rhythm in 31% of cardiac arrests (Gwinnutt *et al.*, 2000). It is an eminently treatable rhythm with most eventual survivors coming from this group (Tunstall-Pedoe *et al.*, 1992). Early defibrillation is the definitive treatment; the chances of success decline substantially with each passing minute (Cobbe *et al.*, 1991). This process can be slowed, but not halted, by effective basic life support (BLS) (Resuscitation Council (UK), 2006).

The Resuscitation Council (UK) ALS algorithm (Figure 8.1) therefore focuses on the need to minimise any delay between the onset of cardiac arrest and defibrillation, if it is required. The algorithm is designed to be an aide-memoire, reminding the practitioner of the important aspects of assessment and treatment of cardiac arrest. It is not designed to be comprehensive or limiting.

Cardiac arrest rhythms can be divided into two groups: shockable (VF/pulseless VT) and non-shockable (pulseless electrical activity (PEA)/asystole). The presenting cardiac arrest rhythm can be classified into one of these two groups and the appropriate pathway in the algorithm then followed. Each step that follows in the algorithm assumes that the previous one has been unsuccessful. Looping the algorithm reinforces the concept of constant reassessment. Apart from defibrillation for the shockable group, the main treatment requirements, e.g. chest compressions, airway management and ventilation, venous access, adrenaline 1 mg intravenously (IV), and the identification and correction of reversible causes, will be common to both groups (Nolan *et al.*, 2005).

Entry into the algorithm depends on the events surrounding the cardiac arrest. If BLS is already in progress, this should continue while the cardiac monitor/defibrillator is attached. Cardiac monitoring provides the link between BLS and ALS. The use of an automated or advisory defibrillator will enable the first responder to defibrillate the patient if necessary prior to the arrival of the cardiac arrest team. If the patient is already on a cardiac monitor, clinical and electrocardiogram (ECG) detection of cardiac arrest will be simultaneous.

It is also important to follow safer handling guidelines (Resuscitation Council (UK), 2001). These are discussed in detail in Chapter 1.

Overview of the ALS algorithm

The procedures described below and the sequences in which they are carried out are based on Resuscitation Council (UK) (2006) recommendations. When more than one healthcare professional is present some of the actions described will be undertaken simultaneously. The main emphasis is on establishing as soon as possible whether defibrillation is required. Guidelines for safe handling during CPR should be followed (Resuscitation Council (UK), 2001).

Unresponsive?

On seeing a patient collapse or when finding a patient who is apparently unconscious, call out for help/pull the emergency buzzer (Figure 8.2), ensure it is safe to approach and proceed to check whether the patient is unresponsive:

- Gently shake the patient's shoulders and ask him loudly 'Are you alright?' (Figure 8.3)

Patient responsive: try to establish the likely cause of the collapse and call for medical assistance. Administer oxygen, start ECG monitoring and secure intravenous access as required.

Patient unresponsive: open the airway and look for signs of life.

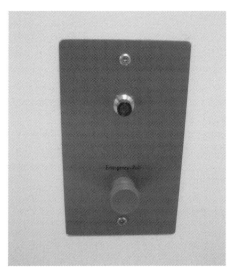

Fig. 8.2 On seeing a patient collapse or when finding a patient who is apparently unconscious, call out for help/pull the emergency buzzer.

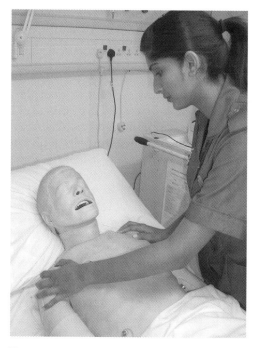

Fig. 8.3 Checking responsiveness: gently shake the shoulders ask loudly 'Are you alright?'

Open the airway and look for signs of life

As the patient is unresponsive and appears to be lifeless, it is important to establish whether he has had a cardiac arrest. Open the airway and look for signs of life:

1. Ideally with the help of colleagues, move the patient into a supine position: if a sliding sheet is already under the patient use that; if not quickly insert one, if possible, under the patient's hips/buttocks by rolling him on to his side and then slide him down the bed (Resuscitation Council (UK), 2001)
2. Leave one pillow *in situ* (helps to maintain a clear airway), but remove all other pillows. If necessary, ask a colleague to remove the backrest
3. Open the airway by tilting the head and lifting the chin (use jaw thrust if trauma to the neck is suspected – see Chapter 6)

4. Ensure the airway is clear.
5. While maintaining the head tilt and chin lift, assess for signs of normal breathing; look for chest movement (breathing or coughing), listen for breath sounds at the patient's mouth and feel for air on your cheek (Soar & Spearpoint, 2005). During the first few minutes following a cardiac arrest the patient may be barely breathing and may be taking infrequent noisy gasps: do not mistake this for normal breathing (Handley *et al.*, 2005). Also look for movement and other signs of life (Resuscitation Council (UK), 2006). Take no longer than 10 seconds to check for signs of normal breathing (Jevon, 2006)
6. If trained to do so, check for the carotid pulse at the same time as checking for signs of normal breathing (Figure 8.4), taking no longer than 10 seconds. Sometimes it can be difficult to establish whether there is a carotid pulse or not (Resuscitation Council (UK), 2006), hence the importance for also assessing for other signs of circulation, e.g. normal breathing and patient movement
7. If the patient is already on an ECG monitor, e.g. on a coronary care unit (CCU), then as well as checking for signs of normal breath/pulse, if able to do so, interpret the ECG to help confirm

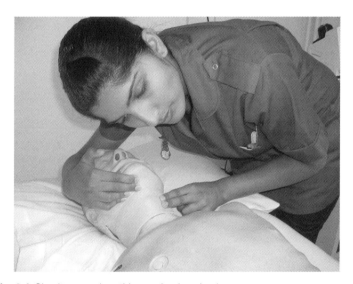

Fig. 8.4 Simultaneous breathing and pulse check.

cardiac arrest. A precordial thump may be appropriate (see below)

Patient breathing normally: ensure the appropriate medical help is on the way. Assess the patient following the ABCDE approach; administer oxygen, commence ECG monitoring and secure intravenous access following local protocols. An unresponsive, but breathing patient should usually be nursed in the lateral position.

Patient not breathing normally/no pulse or if there is any doubt: alert the cardiac arrest team following local protocols and summon/fetch CPR equipment, including the defibrillator. Start CPR 30:2 (if not already, the patient will need to be placed in a supine position, with due regard to safe handling (Resuscitiation Council (UK), 2001)).

If the patient is already on an ECG monitor, is in VF/VT, a defibrillator is immediately at hand and the nurse is trained in manual defibrillation (a scenario commonly occurring on a CCU), defibrillation will should usually be performed immediately, probably without the need for initial CPR.

Call resuscitation team

Call the resuscitation team following local protocols. This usually involves dialling 2222 and telling the telephonist 'Cardiac arrest and location'.

CPR 30:2 until defibrillator/monitor attached

> **A precordial thump, a sharp blow to the patient's sternum with a closed fist, is only recommended when the cardiac arrest is witnessed or monitored and a defibrillator is not immediately at hand (Resuscitation Council (UK), 2006) (see below).**

Start CPR, 30 compressions (see below): two ventilations. While performing chest compressions at a rate of 100 per minute, colleagues should be preparing for ventilation, i.e. inserting an airway device (oropharyngeal airway or laryngeal mask airway

(LMA) (see Chapter 6) and connecting high-flow oxygen to the ventilatory device (e.g. pocket mask or self-inflating bag-mask device (see Chapter 6)). It is important to ensure that a ventilatory device is always immediately available; if one is not available and the nurse is unwilling or it is unsafe to perform mouth-to-mouth ventilation, continue with chest compressions (Soar & Spearpoint, 2005). The techniques for ventilation, including safer handling/ positioning techniques, are discussed in detail in Chapter 6.

Continue CPR while the defibrillator/monitor is being attached. There are three currently used methods (see Chapter 4):

- *ECG leads:* red (right shoulder), yellow (left shoulder) and green (left upper abdominal wall)
- *Defibrillation electrodes/pads:* large, self-adhesive pads, one to the right of the sternum below the clavicle and one over the mid-axillary line approximately level with the V6 ECG electrode position
- *Defibrillator electrodes/paddles:* 'quick look' method using defibrillator paddles enables rapid recognition of a shockable rhythm and prompt defibrillation

Shockable (VF/pulseless VT)

1. If VF/pulseless VT (Figure 8.5a,b) is identified, deliver one shock 150–200 J biphasic (360 J monophasic)

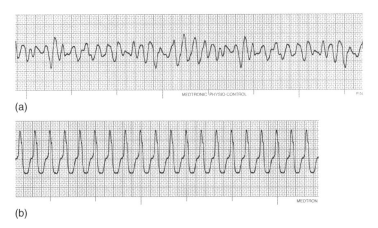

(a)

(b)

Fig. 8.5 (a) VF; (b) pulseless VT. Reproduced with permission from Laerdal Medical Ltd, Orpington, Kent, UK.

2. Recommence (or start) chest compressions 30:2 for 2 minutes without checking the ECG or palpating a pulse
3. After 2 minutes, recheck the ECG and if VF/pulseless VT persists, deliver a second shock 150–360 J biphasic (360 J monophasic)
4. Recommence chest compressions 30:2 for 2 minutes without checking the ECG or palpating a pulse. Prepare adrenaline 1 mg IV
5. After 2 minutes, recheck the ECG and if VF/pulseless VT persists, administer adrenaline 1 mg IV, then deliver a third shock 150–360 J biphasic (360 J monophasic)
6. Recommence chest compressions 30:2 for 2 minutes without checking the ECG or palpating a pulse. Prepare amiodarone 300 mg IV
7. After 2 minutes, recheck the ECG and if VF/pulseless VT persists, administer amiodarone 300 mg IV, then deliver a fourth shock 150–360 J biphasic (360 J monophasic)
8. Continue the 2 minutes CPR/recheck the ECG/defibrillate with 150–360 J biphasic (360 J monophasic) sequence while the patient remains in VF/pulseless VT; administer adrenaline 1 mg IV every 3–5 minutes (i.e. during every other loop)

Pulse checks

Pulse checks (and ECG interpretation) are not recommended following defibrillation (Nolan *et al.*, 2005). It is very rare to be able to palpate a pulse immediately following defibrillation even if a perfusing rhythm is present (Rea *et al.*, 2005); checking for a pulse delays the delivery of chest compressions, further compromising the myocardium if a perfusing rhythm is not present (van Alem *et al.*, 2003). Performing chest compressions in the presence of a perfusing rhythm doesn't increase the risk of another episode of VF; performing chest compressions in the presence of post-shock asystole may actually cause VF (which is helpful) (Hess & White, 2005).

Stopping CPR

It will be necessary to stop CPR while the ECG is interpreted, while defibrillation is undertaken or if the patient shows signs of life.

Shock refractory VF/pulseless VT

In shock refractory VF/pulseless VT, correct any reversible causes, e.g. hypothermia (see below and Chapter 9), as any of these can reduce the likelihood of successful defibrillation (Resuscitation Council (UK), 2006). The anterior–posterior paddle placement for defibrillation and changing defibrillators should also be considered.

Fine VF

If the ECG displays fine VF that is difficult to distinguish from asystole, defibrillation will not be successful and therefore should not be performed because it will increase myocardial damage and interrupt vital chest compressions; instead continue with effective CPR as this may improve the amplitude and frequency of the VF and improve the chance of subsequent successful defibrillation to a perfusing rhythm (Nolan *et al.*, 2005).

Asystole

Following 2 minutes of CPR, if the ECG displayed is asystole (non-shockable) (Figure 8.6), confirm it is asystole (check the leads/connections, check the gain and check the correct monitoring lead on the monitor is selected) and then proceed down the non-shockable (PEA/asystole) side of the algorithm (see below).

Organised electrical activity

Following 2 minutes of CPR, if the ECG displayed is compatible with a pulse, check for a pulse for no longer than 10 seconds. If there is no pulse (PEA), proceed down the non-shockable (PEA/asystole) side of the algorithm (see below). If there is a pulse, perform ABCDE assessment and continue with assisted ventilation if required.

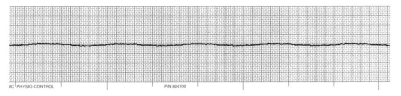

Fig. 8.6 Asystole.

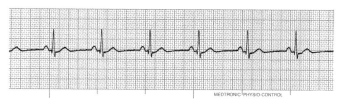

Fig. 8.7 Pulseless electrical activity (PEA).

Non-shockable (PEA/asystole)

PEA

PEA (Figure 8.7) can be defined as organised electrical activity but without a pulse (formerly called electromechanical dissociation (EMD)).

In PEA, mechanical myocardial contractions are usually present, but they are too weak to produce a detectable pulse or blood pressure; it is usually caused by a reversible condition which will need to be identified and effectively treated if the patient is to survive (see below) (Nolan *et al.*, 2005).

The treatment for PEA:

1. Start CPR 30:2
2. Secure the airway as soon as possible so that chest compressions/ventilations can be performed asynchronously
3. Administer adrenaline 1 mg IV as soon as possible and then repeat it every 3–5 minutes (every other loop)
4. If the heart rate <60/minute, administer atropine 3 mg IV once only
5. Identify and treat any reversible causes (see below). A system of checking for and excluding the reversible causes (four Hs and four Ts) is helpful
6. Reassess the ECG trace after 2 minutes; if PEA is still present, check for a pulse. If there is no pulse repeat the above as appropriate. If a pulse is present, assess the patient following the ABCDE approach, providing assisted ventilation as required. If asystole is present, proceed as described below; if VF/pulseless VT is present, and there is no pulse, proceed down the shockable side of the algorithm (see above)

Asystole

It is essential that the correct diagnosis is made. Ensure that the 'straight line' is not being caused by a mechanical problem:

- Ensure the ECG leads are correctly attached
- Ensure the gain (ECG size) is correctly set
- Ensure the correct monitoring lead is selected on the monitor

The treatment for asystole:

1. Carefully check the ECG for P waves (ventricular standstill – Figure 8.8), because this may respond to cardiac pacing (see Principles of external pacing, below) (Nolan *et al.*, 2005)
2. Start CPR 30:2
3. Secure the airway as soon as possible so that chest compressions/ventilations can be performed asynchronously
4. Administer adrenaline 1 mg IV as soon as possible and then repeat it every 3–5 minutes (every other loop)
5. Administer atropine 3 mg IV once only (unless already administered for PEA – see above) (maximum vagal blockade): asystole can be exacerbated or precipitated by excessive vagal tone which theoretically could be reversed by atropine (Nolan *et al.*, 2005)
6. Identify and treat any reversible causes (see below). A system of checking for and excluding the reversible causes (four Hs and four Ts) is helpful
7. Reassess the ECG trace after 2 minutes; if asystole is still present, repeat the above as appropriate. If an organised ECG rhythm is present, check for a pulse. If there is no pulse repeat the above. If a pulse is present, assess the patient following the ABCDE approach, providing assisted ventilation as required.

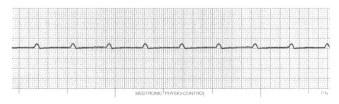

Fig. 8.8 Ventricular standstill. Reproduced with permission from Laerdal Medical Ltd, Orpington, Kent, UK.

If VF/pulseless VT is present, and there is no pulse, proceed down the shockable side of the algorithm (see above)

During cardiopulmonary resuscitation

During the resuscitation attempt, the priorities are to:

- Provide effective chest compressions without interruptions, except for interpretation of the ECG, defibrillation and ventilation when the airway has not yet to be secured
- Defibrillate as required (following the algorithm)
- Secure the airway
- Obtain intravenous access (Figure 8.9)
- Recognise and treat any underlying causes

The ALS algorithm stresses these priorities:

- *Correct reversible causes:* see below
- *Check electrode position and contact:* check and recheck that the ECG trace is reliable

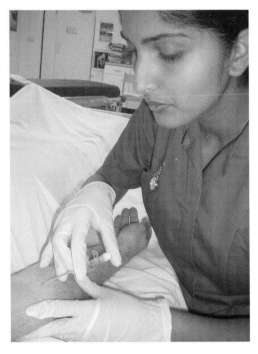

Fig. 8.9 Obtaining intravenous access.

- *Attempt/verify intravenous access, airway and oxygen:* secure intravenous access (depends on expertise, situation and equipment available); secure the airway (see Chapter 6), ideally with a tracheal tube, and ensure that high-flow oxygen is attached – regularly check that the airway is still clear and that the patient is being effectively ventilated with high-flow oxygen
- *Deliver uninterrupted compressions when the airway is secure:* chest compressions and ventilations can be performed asynchronously once the airway is secured with a tracheal tube (this may also be possible if a laryngeal mask has been inserted as long as there is adequate seal pressure around the larynx; however, if excessive gas leakage leads to inadequate lung inflations, a slight pause for ventilation will be required). Chest compressions are tiring: rotate the person undertaking them every few minutes
- *Administer adrenaline every 3–5 minutes:* in a non-shockable rhythm, administer adrenaline 1 mg IV as soon as possible and then repeat it every 3–5 minutes; in a shockable rhythm, adrenaline is delayed until just before the third shock, then repeat it every 3–5 minutes (caution in severe hypothermia – see below and Chapter 9).
- *Consider amiodarone, atropine and magnesium:* consider these drugs in certain situations – see Resuscitation drugs below.

Reversible causes

In every arrest, it is important to identify and treat any reversible causes (four Hs and four Ts). The treatment for these is discussed in detail below.

Chest compressions

The Resuscitation Council (UK) (2006) stresses the importance of chest compressions. On confirmation of cardiac arrest, they should be started immediately while colleagues call the resuscitation team and fetch the cardiac arrest trolley/defibrillator (one exception: if the patient is in VF/VT and defibrillation can be performed immediately by the nurse, e.g. on a CCU, then chest compressions may not be performed prior to defibrillation).

Safer handling techniques

Before starting chest compressions, to minimise the risk of injury it is important to follow Resuscitation Council (UK) (2001) safer handling guidelines:

- Remove any environmental hazards, ensure the bed brakes are on and lower cot sides if they are up
- *Performing chest compressions on a patient on a bed with adjustable height:* ensure the bed is at a height which places the patient between the knee and mid-thigh of the nurse performing chest compressions; stand at the side of the bed with the feet shoulder-width apart, position the shoulders directly over the patient's sternum and keep the arms straight (Figure 8.10). Chest compressions can also be performed by kneeling with both knees on the bed (Figure 8.11)

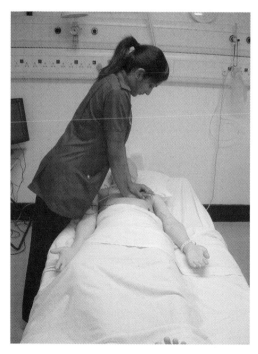

Fig. 8.10 Chest compressions (standing).

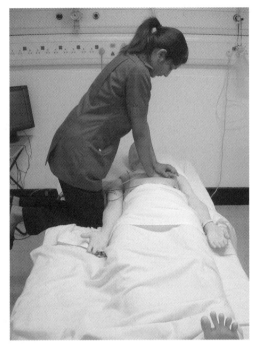

Fig. 8.11 Chest compressions (kneeling on the bed).

- *Performing chest compressions on a patient on a fixed-height bed, couch or trolley:* if necessary, stand on steps or a firm stool, with a non-slip surface and wide enough to permit the nurse's feet to be shoulder-width apart. Position the shoulders directly over the patient's sternum and keep the arms straight; do not kneel on a couch or trolley
- *Performing chest compressions on a patient on the floor:* kneel in the high-kneeling position, at the side of the patient, level with his chest with the knees shoulder-width apart; position the shoulders directly over the patient's sternum and keep the arms straight

Technique

Once the correct position has been adopted (see above):

1. Place the one hand on the centre of the patient's chest (this equates to the middle of the lower half of the sternum) and

then place the other on top (this is a quicker than using the 'rib margin' location method); do not apply pressure over the end of the sternum or the upper abdomen (Handley *et al.*, 2005)

2. Interlock and extend the fingers to avoid applying pressure over the patient's ribs
3. Apply pressure to the sternum only; do not apply pressure to the ribs, the end of the sternum or the upper abdomen (Handley *et al.*, 2005)
4. Position the shoulders directly vertical above the patient's sternum, straighten the arms and lock the elbows; ensure the back is not twisted
5. Compress the sternum 4–5 cm and, following each compression, allow the chest to completely recoil back to its normal position (Yannopoulos *et al.*, 2005), thus facilitating venous return
6. Ensure that the force of compression results from flexing the hips (Resuscitation Council (UK), 2001)
7. Perform chest compressions in a controlled manner; they should not be erratic or jerky (Jevon, 2006)
8. Continue chest compressions at a rate of 100/minute; this rate refers to the speed of compressions rather than the actual number delivered per minute; interruptions in chest compressions, e.g. to allow defibrillation, will result in less than 100 being delivered in a minute
9. Ensure that the chest compression/chest relaxation phases are of equal duration
10. Ensure a ratio of 30 compressions: two ventilations (30:2) to allow more time for chest compressions (asynchronous once the patient has a secure airway)
11. To prevent fatigue, rotate the person performing chest compressions approximately every 2 minutes (Nolan *et al.*, 2005)

It is important to follow Resuscitation Council (UK) (2001) safer handling guidelines during CPR (see above). Ventilate using available airway and ventilation devices. Once the defibrillator arrives apply ECG leads/defibrillation pads and, if indicated, defibrillate immediately if trained to do so.

Mechanical chest compression devices

Even if performed effectively, the standard technique for chest compressions only achieves 30% of normal cardiac output

(Del Guercio *et al.*, 1965). Several mechanical chest compression devices (Figure 8.12) have been developed to attempt to improve circulation during CPR; to date, no adjunct has consistently been shown to be superior to conventional manual CPR (Nolan *et al.*, 2005).

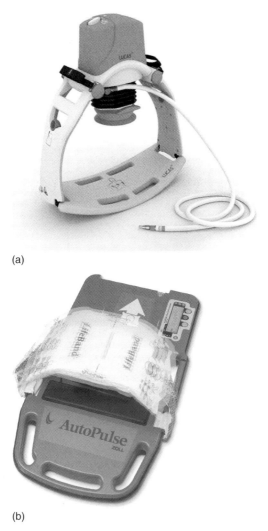

(a)

(b)

Fig. 8.12 Mechanical chest compression devices. Reproduced with permission of (a) Medtronic Ltd, Watford, UK, and (b) Zoll Medical UK Ltd, Runcorn, UK.

Precordial thump

The precordial thump is a blow to the lower half of the patient's sternum using the lateral aspect of a closed fist (Jevon, 2006). It can successfully resuscitate the patient, when given promptly following a cardiac arrest caused by VF/VT (Resuscitation Council (UK), 2006).

Mechanism of action

The rationale for delivering a precordial thump is that it generates a mechanical energy which is converted to electrical energy which then may be sufficient to achieve successful cardioversion (Kohl *et al.*, 2005). Following the onset of VF, the threshold for successful defibrillation rises steeply after a few seconds. In all reported cases of successful use of the precordial thump for VF, it was delivered within 10 seconds (Resuscitation Council (UK), 2006). Hence the importance of witnessing the collapse.

Indications

A precordial thump should be considered if cardiac arrest is confirmed rapidly following a witnessed and monitored (ECG) sudden collapse (VF/VT), if the defibrillator is not immediately at hand (Resuscitation Council (UK), 2006).

Efficacy

In 187 episodes of VF, VT, supraventricular tachycardia, asystole and complete heart block where a precordial thump was delivered:

- 91 (49%) reverted to normal sinus rhythm
- 77 (41%) had no change in rhythm
- 19 (10%) became worse
- Overall: 90% of patients were either better or no change and 10% were worse

(American Heart Association, 2006)

Procedure

A precordial thump should be considered if cardiac arrest is confirmed rapidly following a witnessed and monitored (ECG) sudden collapse (VF/VT), if the defibrillator is not immediately at hand (Resuscitation Council (UK), 2006):

1. Tightly clench the fist (the dominant hand is usually used)
2. Position the fist approximately 20 cm directly above the patient's sternum
3. Using the ulnar edge of the fist, deliver a sharp blow to the lower half of the sternum (Resuscitation Council (UK), 2006) (Figure 8.13). An effective, but not excessive, force, can be generated by swinging the fist from the elbow (Adam & Osborne, 2005)
4. Immediately then retract the fist to create an impulse-like stimulus (Nolan *et al.*, 2005)
5. Prepare to start CPR (30 compressions: two ventilations) (Resuscitation Council (UK), 2006). If the precordial thump successfully terminates VF/VT, it is probable that the patient will regain consciousness very quickly, sometimes almost spontaneously, i.e. CPR will therefore not be required

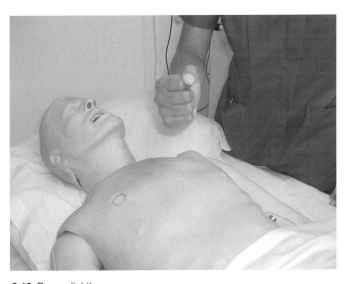

Fig. 8.13 Precordial thump.

Complications

There are isolated cases reported in the literature of a precordial thump converting a pulse-producing rhythm to a non-pulse-producing rhythm (Krijne, 1984), though this is a very rare phenomenon (Resuscitation Council (UK), 2006). There is also a risk of damaging the ribcage, particularly if the precordial thump is incorrectly delivered. Nevertheless, the potential benefit of the precordial thump greatly outweighs its risks (Caldwell *et al.*, 1985).

Reversible causes

The search for, and treatment of, potential reversible causes of cardiac arrest is paramount, particularly when PEA is present. Clues to the possible cause of cardiopulmonary arrest may be obtained by checking the history and undertaking a physical examination; aggressive treatment of an identified reversible cause is paramount in order to restore coronary perfusion pressure and spontaneous circulation (Aufderheide *et al.*, 2007).

The potential reversible causes can conveniently be classified into two groups for ease of memory – four Hs and four Ts and will now be briefly discussed.

Hypoxia: causes such as asphyxiation, e.g. foreign body aspiration, and strangulation may be obvious after checking the history and clinical examination; other causes of hypoxia include existing respiratory disease, e.g. chronic obstructive pulmonary disease (COPD) and asthma, tension pneumothorax and pulmonary embolism (Aufderheide *et al.*, 2007); if hypoxia is suspected, secure the airway with a tracheal tube, and ventilate with 100% oxygen, checking that there is bilateral air entry.

Hypovolaemia: this is the main cause of PEA in approximately 4–5% of pre-hospital cardiac arrests (Stueven *et al.*, 1989); it is usually caused by severe haemorrhage. The priority is to restore intravascular volume with appropriate fluids to ensure adequate preload (Aufderheide *et al.*, 2007); if necessary, arrange urgent surgery to stop the bleeding.

Hyperkalaemia/hypokalaemia and metabolic disorders: this diagnosis is confirmed by laboratory tests, though the patient's history, e.g. renal failure, could indicate possible abnormal blood chemistry. Abnormalities should be corrected as appropriate. Administer calcium chloride 10% 10 ml IV if hyperkalaemia, hypocalcaemia or an overdose of calcium channel blockers is suspected or confirmed.

Hypothermia: this should be particularly suspected following an immersion injury. Use a low reading thermometer and rapidly rewarm the patient, e.g. warm intravenous fluids, warm humidified air via a tracheal tube, extracorporeal cardiopulmonary bypass (Aufderheide *et al.*, 2007). In addition, as CPR is often required for prolonged periods, it is recommended to use a mechanical chest compression device to enable consistent delivery of effective chest compressions (Wik & Kiil, 2005). See Chapter 9 for further information relating to CPR in hypothermic patients.

Tension pneumothorax: incidence of tension pneumothorax may be as high as 4% of PEA cardiac arrests (Jevon, 2002). It is suggested by unilateral decreased breath sounds following tracheal intubation, distended jugular veins, tracheal deviation away from the affected side and hyper-resonnance to percussion over the affected side (Aufderheide *et al.*, 2007). Causes include chest trauma, asthma, central venous cannulation and mechanical ventilation.

The emergency treatment is initially needle thoracentesis followed by insertion of a chest drain. Aufderheide *et al.* (2007) recommend the following procedure for needle thoracentesis:

1. If possible quickly prepare the insertion site using an iodine-based solution
2. Briefly suspend CPR while the procedure is undertaken
3. Insert a size 14–18 gauge catheter in the second intercostal space, mid-clavicular line on the affected side
4. Once the pleural space is entered, advance the catheter over the needle
5. Remove the needle and aspirate air using a syringe

6. Attach a three-way tap to the catheter to allow repeated aspiration of air as necessary (Ross, 1998)

Tamponade: cardiac tamponade occurs when blood or other fluid fills the pericardial space, raising intrapericardial pressure, compressing the heart and preventing it from filling (Jevon, 2002). An uncommon cause of cardiac arrest, it can occur in patients with cancer, recent cardiothoracic surgery, coagulopathy, platelet disorder or chest trauma (Aufderheide *et al.*, 2007). Clinical features include distended neck veins, hypotension and muffled heart sounds; unfortunately, these can be obscured by the cardiac arrest itself. Initially perform needle pericardiocentisis to relieve the tamponade. Aufderheide *et al.* (2007) recommend the following procedure for needle pericardiocentisis:

1. Quickly prepare the subxiphoid region using an iodine-based solution
2. Briefly suspend CPR while the procedure is undertaken
3. Insert a size 16–18 gauge catheter between the xiphoid process and the left subcostal angle at a 30–45 degree angle to the chest; the needle should be directed towards the inferior tip of the patient's left scapula
4. Once fluid is aspirated, advance the catheter into the pericardial space, remove the needle and attach a three-way tap (Bartlett, 1998)

Thromboembolic or mechanical circulatory obstruction: if a pulmonary embolism is suspected, an emergency pulmonary embolectomy is the definitive treatment and can be life-saving; if possible the patient should be transferred to a cardiovascular surgical department. Practically, in most healthcare settings, emergency pulmonary embolectomy will not be feasible. However, the immediate administration of a thrombolytic drug should be considered (Bottiger *et al.*, 2001).

Toxic/therapeutic disturbances: if there is no specific history related to toxic or therapeutic disturbances, the cause may only be established following laboratory investigations. If applicable, administer the appropriate antidote. Treatment is often only supportive.

Drug delivery routes

Intravenous

The intravenous route remains the most reliable for drug administration during resuscitation (Resuscitation Council (UK), 2006). If the patient already has a cannula *in situ*, which has been confirmed patent, use it first (Resuscitation Council (UK), 2006).

If intravenous access needs to be obtained, the route selected will depend on the expertise and experience of the operator and the availability of equipment (Resuscitation Council (UK), 2006). The peripheral route, e.g. anti-cubital fossa, is usually the preferred option because it is least invasive, is associated with a low risk of complications and cannula insertion shouldn't hinder CPR. However, peripherally injected drugs should be flushed into the central circulation using intravenous fluid (Nolan *et al.*, 2005) and the limb should be elevated (Emerman *et al.*, 1988).

The central route, e.g. subclavian or internal jugular, can provide higher drug concentrations and has minimal circulation time. Unfortunately it can be difficult to establish, can interrupt CPR and complications can be life threatening, e.g. air embolism. Therefore practically, if intravenous access needs to be obtained during resuscitation, the peripheral route is usually selected (Jevon, 2007).

When administering a drug intravenously during CPR:

1. Ask a colleague to check the drug – name of drug, dose, strength and expiry date following Nursing and Midwifery Council (NMC) (2008) guidelines
2. Administer the drug intravenously (ideally via a central venous catheter, though in practice it will usually be a peripheral cannula)
3. Flush with a minimum of 20 ml of fluid; it is the policy at some healthcare establishments to set up an intravenous infusion for this purpose ('chaser fluid')
4. Elevate the limb for 10–20 seconds to facilitate drug delivery to the central circulation (Emerman *et al.*, 1988)

Intraosseous

The intraosseous route is an option if intravenous access can not be established (Nolan *et al.*, 2005). Traditionally used in infants

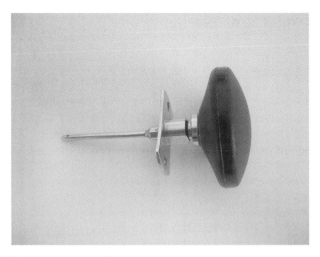

Fig. 8.14 Intraosseous needle.

and children (Jevon, 2003), intraosseous access is safe and effective in adults (Macnab *et al.*, 2000). The two best sites are the proximal tibia and distal tibia (Resuscitation Council (UK), 2006). Intraosseous access is suitable for drug administration, but not fluid resuscitation (Resuscitation Council (UK), 2006). A standard intraosseous needle is depicted in Figure 8.14.

When administering a drug intraosseously during CPR:

1. Ask a colleague to check the drug – name of drug, dose, strength and expiry date following NMC (2008) guidelines
2. Administer the drug intraosseously and then flush with a minimum of 20 ml of fluid

Tracheal tube

The tracheal tube route can be considered if intravenous or intraosseous access is delayed or can not be secured (Nolan *et al.*, 2005). Resuscitation drugs that can be administered via this route include adrenaline and atropine (Jevon, 2007). Absorption is variable and higher doses of the drug need to be administered in order to be able to achieve desired plasma concentrations (Hornchen *et al.*, 1987). The drug should be diluted with sterile water, not 0.9% normal saline (Naganobu *et al.*, 2000); a total volume of 10–20 ml is currently recommended (Resuscitation Council (UK), 2006).

When administering a drug via the tracheal tube:

1. Ask a colleague to check the drug (and sterile water) – name of drug, dose, strength and expiry date following NMC (2008) guidelines
2. Prepare the recommended dose. The dose of adrenaline via this route is 3 mg diluted to at least 10 ml with sterile water (Resuscitation Council (UK), 2005)
3. Disconnect the bag–mask device from the tracheal tube
4. Administer the drug into the tracheal tube; ventilations will then disperse the drug into the lungs

(Jevon, 2007)

Intracardiac

Intracardiac injection (i.e. injection directly into the ventricles) is no longer recommended because it can be difficult to perform, may interrupt resuscitation and carries a high risk of complications, e.g. laceration of the coronary artery, pneumothorax (Jevon, 2002).

Resuscitation drugs

A few drugs are indicated during the initial management of a cardiac arrest, though scientific evidence to support their use is limited (Nolan *et al.*, 2005). They can be considered once defibrillation has been performed (if indicated) and CPR has been started (Jevon, 2007).

Adrenaline

Adrenaline is first drug administered during CPR. Its main benefit is to improve coronary and cerebral blood flow (Jevon, 2002). The dose is 1 mg (10 ml of 1:10 000 solution) IV, repeated every 3–5 minutes (Nolan *et al.*, 2005). If the tracheal route is used the dose is 3 mg (3 ml of 1:1000 solution) made up with sterile water to a volume of 10 ml (Resuscitation Council (UK), 2006).

Amiodarone

Amiodarone is the preferred anti-arrhythmic drug for use in CPR. It is administered if the patient remains in VF/pulseless VT despite three defibrillatory shocks (Nolan *et al.*, 2005). The initial dose is 300 mg IV, diluted with 5% dextrose to a volume of 20 ml (or use a pre-filled syringe format).

When administered peripherally, amiodarone can cause thrombophlebitis. Ideally it should therefore be administered via a central venous catheter, though if one is not *in situ*, a large peripheral vein can be used followed by a flush (Nolan *et al.*, 2005). The once popular anti-arrhythmic drug lignocaine should only be used if amiodarone is not available.

Magnesium sulphate

Magnesium sulphate is indicated in refractory VF if hypomagnesaemia is suspected, e.g. hypokalaemia. The recommended dose is 8 mmol (4 ml of 50% solution) IV (or intraosseously) administered over 1–2 minutes; it may be repeated after 10–15 minutes (Nolan *et al.*, 2005).

Atropine

Atropine antagonises the action of the vagus nerve and is indicated in asystole and in PEA) when the QRS rate <60/minute (Jevon, 2007). During CPR, the recommended dose is 3 mg IV (or intraosseously), administered once only.

Calcium

Calcium is indicated during CPR for PEA if it has been caused by hyperkalaemia, hypocalcaemia, overdose of calcium channel blockers or overdose of magnesium (e.g. during the treatment of eclampsia) (Resuscitation Council (UK), 2005). It is required for myocardial contraction, though high plasma concentrations can have detrimental effects on the ischaemic myocardium and may impair cerebral recovery (Nolan *et al.*, 2005).

The recommended initial dose is 10 ml of 10% calcium chloride IV (or intraosseously), repeated if necessary. Careful administration is required as extravasion around the cannula can cause severe tissue injury; it should not administered simultaneously with sodium bicarbonate via the same route as this will result in calcium carbonate (chalk) formation (Jevon, 2007).

Sodium bicarbonate

Following a cardiac arrest, anaerobic cellular metabolism and the cessation of pulmonary gas exchange cause metabolic and respiratory acidosis respectively. Sodium bicarbonate has traditionally been used in CPR to 'correct' this acidosis. However there are numerous detrimental side effects, including generation of carbon dioxide, exacerbation of intracellular acidosis and inhibition of oxygen release to the tissues (Resuscitation Council (UK), 2006).

The optimum treatment for acidosis is effective ventilation and chest compressions, which in previously healthy individuals, is normally quite sufficient to prevent a rapid or severe development of acidosis (Jevon, 2002).

The routine use of sodium bicarbonate is not recommended; it is indicated if the cardiac arrest is associated with hyperkalaemia or tricyclic anti-depressant overdose (Nolan *et al.*, 2005). The dose is 50 mmol IV (50 ml of 8.4% solution). Some authorities recommend sodium bicarbonate if severe metabolic acidosis (pH < 7.1 and base excess <−10) is present; however this is controversial (Resuscitation Council (UK), 2006).

Lignocaine

Lignocaine should be considered in refractory VF/VT, when the first three defibrillatory shocks have been unsuccessful and when amiodarone is unavailable (Jevon, 2007). The dose is 100 mg IV (5 ml of 2% solution); a further 50 mg IV may be required.

Use of pre-filled syringes

There are two main pre-filled syringe products for drug administration during CPR. The use of both will be described.

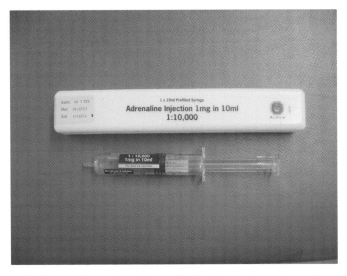

Fig. 8.15 Remove the cap from the pre-filled syringe and expel any air.

Preparation of product 1 (Figure 8.15)

1. Check the details of the drug on the pre-filled syringe box
2. Open the pre-filled syringe box by using a slight twisting action
3. Remove the pre-filled syringe, and check the drug details including name, dose and expiry date
4. Remove the cap from the pre-filled syringe and expel any air. It is now ready for use (Figure 8.15)

(Source: Jevon, 2007)

Preparation of product 2 (Figures 8.16 and 8.17)

1. Check the details of the drug on the pre-filled syringe box
2. Open the pre-filled syringe box by ripping the one end off as indicated
3. Remove the vial and syringe barrel and check the drug details on the vial including name, dose and expiry date on
4. Remove the cap from the vial and the lower end of the syringe barrel (Figure 8.16)

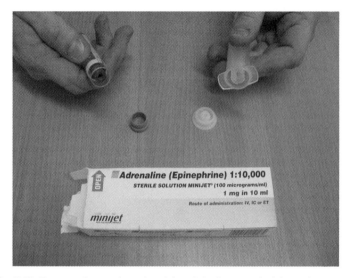

Fig. 8.16 Remove the cap from the vial and the lower end of the syringe barrel.

5. Thread the vial into the syringe barrel, turning it 3.5 times; resistance will now be met
6. Remove the cap from the top of the syringe barrel and expel any air. It is now ready for use (Figure 8.17)

(Jevon, 2007)

Principles of external pacing

Cardiac pacing is the delivery of a small electrical current to the heart to stimulate myocardial contraction. External (transcutaneous or percussion) pacing can be established quickly and easily during CPR. It buys time for the spontaneous recovery of the conduction system or for more definitive treatment to be established, e.g. transvenous pacing.

Indications

- *Profound bradycardia:* sometimes found in complete heart block, that has not responded to pharmacological treatment,

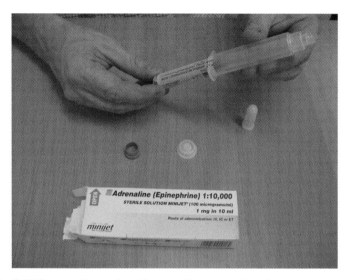

Fig. 8.17 Remove the cap from the top of the syringe barrel and expel any air. It is now ready for use.

e.g. atropine. N.B. if the intrinsic QRS complexes are not associated with a pulse (PEA), attempts at pacing will be futile

- *Ventricular standstill:* P waves (atrial contraction) only on the ECG (Figure 8.8)

N.B. Although pacing is not indicated in asystole, always carefully check the ECG for the presence of P waves (ventricular standstill) as this may respond to pacing (Nolan *et al.*, 2005).

Advantages of trancutaneous pacing

- Can be quickly established
- Easy to undertake, minimal training
- Risks associated with central venous cannulation are avoided
- Can be undertaken by nurses

(Resuscitation Council (UK), 2006)

Procedure for transcutaneous pacing

1. If appropriate, explain the procedure to the patient
2. Ideally, first remove excess chest hair from the pacing electrode sites by clipping close to the patient's skin using a pair

of scissors (shaving the skin is not recommended as any nicks in the skin can lead to burns and pain during pacing) (Resuscitation Council (UK), 2006)

3. Attach the pacing electrodes following the manufacturer's instructions:
   - Pacing-only electrodes: attach the anterior electrode on the left anterior chest, midway between the xiphoid process and the left nipple (V2–V3 ECG electrode position) and attach the posterior electrode below the left scapula, lateral to the spine and at the same level as the anterior electrode – this anterior/posterior configuration will ensure that the position of the electrodes does not interfere with defibrillation (Resuscitation Council (UK), 2006). ECG monitoring will usually need to be established if an older pacing system is used (Resuscitation Council (UK), 2006)
   - Multifunctional electrodes (pacing and defibrillation): place the anterior electrode below the right clavicle and the lateral electrode in the mid-axillary line lateral to the left nipple (V6 ECG electrode position) – this anterior–lateral position is convenient during CPR as chest compressions do not have to be interrupted (Resuscitation Council (UK), 2006)

4. Check that the pacing electrodes and connecting cables are applied following the manufacturer's recommendations: if they are reversed, pacing may either be ineffective or high capture thresholds may be required (Resuscitation Council (UK), 2006)

5. Adjust the ECG gain (size) accordingly. This will help ensure that the intrinsic QRS complexes are sensed

6. Select demand mode on the pacing unit on the defibrillator

7. Select an appropriate rate for external pacing, usually 60–90/minute

8. Set the pacing current at the lowest level, turn on the pacemaker unit and while observing both the patient and the ECG, gradually increase the current until electrical capture occurs (QRS complexes following the pacing spike) (Jevon, 2002). Electrical capture usually occurs when the current delivered is in the range of 50–100 mA (Resuscitation Council (UK), 2006)

9. Check the patient's pulse. If he has a palpable pulse (mechanical capture), request expert help and prepare for transvenous pacing. If there is no pulse, start CPR. If there is good electrical capture, but no mechanical capture, this is indicative of a non-

viable myocardium (Resuscitation Council (UK), 2006). N.B. there is no electrical hazard if in contact with the patient during pacing (Resuscitation Council (UK), 2006)

(Jevon, 2007)

Cautions

- If the patient is conscious, analgesia and sedation will usually be required
- If pacing-only electrodes have been applied and defibrillation is subsequently indicated, position the defibrillation paddles least 2–3 cm away from the pacing electrodes to avoid arcing
- Turn off pacemaker unit during CPR to prevent inappropriate stimulation of the patient (Resuscitation Council (UK), 2006)

Percussion pacing

Percussion pacing can result in a cardiac output with minimal trauma to the patient. It is likely to be successful when there is ventricular standstill (P waves, but no QRS complexes). It involves the delivery of gentle blows (from a height of only a few inches above the chest) over the precordium lateral to the lower left sternal edge (Resuscitation Council (UK), 2006). Trial and error will determine the optimum place for percussion.

Chapter summary

ALS is the term used to describe the more specialised techniques employed to support breathing and circulation during CPR, as well as specific treatment used to try and restore cardiac output. In this chapter, an overview of ALS has been provided with specific reference to the Resuscitation Council (UK) ALS algorithm.

References

Adam S, Osborne S (2005) *Critical Care Nursing Science and Practice*, 2nd Ed. Oxford University Press, Oxford.

American Heart Association (2006) *Worksheet BLS – Alternative methods of CPR including cough CPR and precordial thump (B)*. www.americanheart.org (accessed 4 April 2009)

Aufderheide T, Larabee T, Paradis N (2007) Special considerations in the therapy of non-fibrillatory cardiac arrest. In: Paradis N *et al.* (Eds) *Cardiac Arrest: The Science and Practice of Resuscitation Medicine*, 2nd Ed. Cambridge University Press, Cambridge.

Bartlett R (1998) Resuscitative thoracotomy. In: Roberts J, Hedges J (Eds) *Clinical Procedures in Emergency Medicine*. WB Saunders, Philadelphia.

Bottiger B, Bode C, Kern S *et al.* (2001) Efficacy and safety of thrombolytic therapy after initially unsuccessful resuscitation: a prospective clinical trial. *Lancet* **357**:1583–5.

Caldwell G, Millar G, Quinn E *et al.* (1985) Simple mechanical methods for cardioversion: defence of the precordial thump and cough version. *British Medical Journal* **291**:627–30.

Cobbe S, Redmond M, Watson J *et al.* (1991) Heartstart Scotland – initial experience of a national scheme for out of hospital defibrillation. *British Medical Journal* **302**:1517–20.

Del Guercio LRM, Feins NR, Cohn JD *et al.* (1965) Comparison of blood flow during external and internal cardiac massage in man. *Circulation* **31**(Suppl. 1):1171–80.

Emerman C, Pinchak A, Hancock D, Hagen J (1988) Effect of injection site on circulation times during cardiac arrest. *Critical Care Medicine* **16**:1138–41.

Gwinnutt C, Columb M, Harris R (2000) Outcome after cardiac arrest in adults in UK hospitals: effect of the 1997 guidelines. *Resuscitation* **47**:125–35.

Handley A, Koster R, Monsieurs K *et al.* (2005) European Resuscitation Council Guidelines for Resuscitation 2005: Section 2. Adult basic life support and use of automated external defibrillators. *Resuscitation* **67S1**:S7–S23.

Hess E, White R (2005) Ventricular fibrillation is not provoked by chest compression during post-shock organized rhythms in out-of-hospital cardiac arrest. *Resuscitation* **66**:7–11.

Hornchen U, Schuttler J, Stoeckel H *et al.* (1987) Endobronchial instillation of epinephrine during cardiopulmonary resuscitation. *Critical Care Medicine* **15**:1037–9.

Jevon P (2002) *Advanced Cardiac Life Support*. Butterworth Heinemann, Oxford.

Jevon P (2003) *Paediatric Advanced Life Support*. Elsevier, London.

Jevon P (2006) Cardiopulmonary resuscitation: chest compressions. *Nursing Times* **98**(22):47–8.

Jevon P (2007) The administration of drugs during resuscitation. *Nursing Times* **103**(11):26–7.

Krijne R (1984) Rate acceleration of ventricular tachycardia after a precordial chest thump. *American Journal of Cardiology* **53**:964–5.

Kohl P, King A, Boulin C (2005) Antiarrhythmic effects of acute mechanical stimulation. In: Kohl P *et al.* (Eds) *Cardiac Mechano-Electric Feedback and Arrhythmias from Pipette to Patient*. Elseveir Saunders, Philadelphia.

Macnab A, Christenson J, Findlay J (2000) A new system for sternal intraosseous infusion in adults. *Prehospital Emergency Care* **4**:173–7.

Naganobu K, Hasebe Y, Uchiyama Y *et al.* (2000) A comparison of distilled water and normal saline as dilutents for endobronchial administration of epinephrine in the dog. *Anesthesia & Analgesia* **91**:317–21.

Nolan J, Deakin C, Soar J *et al.* (2005) European Resuscitation Council Guidelines for Resuscitation 2005: Section 4. Adult advanced life support. *Resuscitation* **675S**:S39–S86.

Nursing and Midwifery Council (2008) *The Code.* NMC, London.

Rea T, Shah S, Kudenchuk P *et al.* (2005) Automated external defibrillators: to what extent does the algorithm delay CPR? *Annals of Emergency Medicine* **46**:132–41.

Resuscitation Council (UK) (2001) *Guidance for Safer Handling During Resuscitation in Hospitals.* Resuscitation Council (UK), London.

Resuscitation Council (UK) (2005) *Resuscitation Guidelines 2005.* Resuscitation Council (UK), London.

Resuscitation Council (UK) (2006) *Advanced Life Support*, 5th Ed. Resuscitation Council (UK), London.

Ross D (1998) Thoracentesis. In: Roberts J, Hedges J (Eds) *Clinical Procedures in Emergency Medicine.* WB Saunders, Philadelphia.

Soar J, Spearpoint K (2005) In-hospital resuscitation. In: *Resuscitation Guidelines 2005.* Resuscitation Council (UK), London.

Stueven H, Aufderheide T, Waite E, Mateer J (1989) Electromechanical dissociation: six years per-hospital experience. *Resuscitation* **17**:173–82.

Tunstall-Pedoe H, Bailey L, Chamberlain D *et al.* (1992) Survey of 3765 cardiopulmonary resuscitations in British hospitals (the BRESUS study): methods and overall results. *British Medical Journal* **304**: 1347–51.

van Alem A, Sanou B, Koster R (2003) Interruption of cardiopulmonary resuscitation with the use of the automated external defibrillator in out-of-hospital cardiac arrest. *Annals of Emergency Medicine* **42**: 449–57.

Wik L, Kiil S (2005) Use of an automatic chest compression device (LUCAS) as a bridge to establishing cardiopulmonary bypass for a patient with hypothermic cardiac arrest. *Resuscitation* **66**:391–4.

Yannopoulos D, McKnite S, Aufderheide T *et al.* (2005) Effects of incomplete chest wall decompression during cardiopulmonary resuscitation on coronary and cerebral perfusion pressures in a porcine model of cardiac arrest. *Resuscitation* **64**: 363–72.

Chapter 9

Resuscitation in Special Situations

Introduction

Resuscitation in certain special situations, e.g. late pregnancy, requires modification to the standard Resuscitation Council (UK) advanced life support (ALS) guidelines (Resuscitation Council (UK), 2006), described in Chapter 8, in order to optimise the chances of survival.

The special situations described in this chapter account for a large proportion of cardiopulmonary arrests in younger persons. As there is often no co-existing cardiorespiratory disease, prognosis is relatively good as long as effective cardiopulmonary resuscitation (CPR) is instigated promptly (Resuscitation Council (UK), 2006). However, if the signs and symptoms are recognised early and effective treatment instigated, cardiac arrest may be prevented (Resuscitation Council (UK), 2006).

The aim of this chapter is to understand the principles of resuscitation in special situations.

Learning outcomes

At the end of the chapter the reader will be able to discuss the principles of resuscitation associated with the following special situations:

- Life-threatening electrolyte abnormalities
- Hypothermia
- Submersion
- Acute severe asthma
- Electrocution
- Late pregnancy

- Poisoning
- Trauma
- Local anaesthetic toxicity

Life-threatening electrolyte abnormalities

Life-threatening electrolyte abnormalities, e.g. hypokalaemia and hyperkalaemia, can cause cardiac arrhythmias and cardiac arrest.

Hyperkalaemia

Hyperkalaemia can be defined as a serum potassium >5.5 mmol/l (Wyatt *et al.*, 2006). Causes include:

- Renal failure leading to a fall in potassium excretion
- Drugs, e.g. angiotensin converting enzyme (ACE) inhibitors, potassium-sparing diuretics (e.g. amiloride)
- Cell injury, e.g. crush injury and rhabdomyolysis
- Following a massive blood transfusion
(Soar *et al.*, 2005; Wyatt *et al.*, 2006)

Hyperkalaemia should be excluded in all patients with a cardiac arrhythmia or cardiac arrest. Electrocardiogram (ECG) abnormalities are common, particularly if serum potassium >6.7 mmol/l.

Depending on the severity of hyperkalaemia, the aims of treatment are to:

- Protect the myocardium
- Move potassium into the cells
- Remove potassium from the body
- Monitor serum potassium levels in case rebound hypokalaemia occurs
- Prevent recurrence
(Soar *et al.*, 2005)

Treatment for hyperkalaemia in a patient not in cardiac arrest
Treatment will depend on the severity of the hyperkalaemia and whether toxic electrocardiogram (ECG) ECG changes are present:

- If the patient is hypovolaemic, administer fluids to enhance renal potassium secretion
- If potassium is 5.5–6 mmol/l (mild elevation), remove potassium from the body: strategies include calcium resonium (potassium exchange resin) 15–30 g orally or retention enema, intravenous furosemide 1 mg/kg and dialysis
- If potassium is 6–6.5 mmol/l (moderate elevation) but without ECG changes, move potassium into the cells: 10 units of short acting insulin in 50 g glucose IV over 15–30 minutes, as well as the above 'potassium removal' strategies
- If potassium is 6.5 mmol/l or more (severe elevation) but without ECG changes, move potassium into the cells: salbutamol 5 mg via nebuliser (a few doses may be required), sodium bicarbonate 50 mmol IV over 5 mins if metabolic acidosis is present and glucose/insulin (see above); also use 'potassium removal' strategies (see above)
- If potassium is 6.5 mmol/l or more with toxic ECG changes (severe elevation), protect the myocardium and reduce the risk of ventricular fibrillation (VF) with calcium chloride 10% 10 ml IV over 2–3 minutes; also use 'potassium removal', and 'moving potassium into the cells' strategies described above

(Soar *et al.*, 2005; Resuscitation Council (UK), 2006)

Treatment for hyperkalaemia in a patient in cardiac arrest
There are no modifications to basic life support (BLS) and ALS; the general approach to treatment will be depend on the severity of the hyperkalaemia, the rate and rise of serum potassium and the patient's clinical condition (Soar *et al.*, 2005).

There are two key priorities: to protect the myocardium and to lower the serum potassium levels by shifting and removal strategies:

- *Protect the myocardium*: administer 10 ml of calcium chloride 10% IV (rapid bolus injection) to antagonise the toxic effects of hyperkalaemia at the myocardial cell membrane
- *Shifting strategy*: if there is severe hyperkalaemia or renal failure, rapidly administer 50 mmol of sodium bicarbonate IV
- *Removal strategies*: rapidly administer dextrose/insulin IV (10 units of short acting insulin and 50 g glucose); consider haemodialysis if medical treatment has failed (consider it

early if there is established renal failure, oliguric renal failure or where marked tissue breakdown is present)

(Resuscitation Council (UK), 2006)

Hypokalaemia

Hypokalaemia can be defined as a serum potassium <3.5 mmol/l (Wyatt *et al.*, 2006) and is common in hospitalised patients (Rastegar & Soleimani, 2001).

Causes
Causes include:

- Diarrhoea leading to gastrointestinal loss
- Drugs, e.g. diuretics, steroids and laxatives
- Endocrine disorders, e.g. Cushing's syndrome
- Metabolic acidosis
- Hypomagnesaemia
- Dialysis

(Soar *et al.*, 2005; British Medical Association & Royal Pharmaceutical Society of Great Britain, 2008)

Hypokalaemia should be excluded in all patients with a cardiac arrhythmia or cardiac arrest (Niemann & Cairns, 1999). ECG abnormalities that may be evident in the presence of hypokalaemia include:

- U waves
- Flattened T waves
- ST segment changes
- Cardiac arrhythmias
- Cardiopulmonary arrest

(Resuscitation Council (UK), 2006)

Treatment
Gradual administration of oral potassium is preferable. However, in the emergency situation intravenous potassium will be required. Although the maximum recommended dose of potassium is 1020 mmol over 1 hour, if the patient has unstable cardiac

arrhythmias and cardiac arrest is imminent or indeed has occurred, potassium 20 mmol IV over 10 minutes (2 mmol/per minute) followed by potassium 5–10 mmol over 5–10 minutes is recommended (Soar *et al.*, 2005; Resuscitation Council (UK), 2006).

Hypomagnesaemia is often associated with hypokalaemia (magnesium is important for the uptake of potassium and for the maintenance of intracellular potassium levels) (Soar *et al.*, 2005). It is therefore recommended to replenish magnesium stores if hypokalaemia is severe (Cohn *et al.*, 2000).

Hypercalcaemia, hypocalcaemia, hypermagnesaemia and hypomagnesaemia

The recognition and emergency treatment of calcium and magnesium disorders are detailed in Table 9.1.

Hypothermia

Hypothermia can mimic death and death can mimic hypothermia.

(Bowden, 2001)

Hypothermia can be defined as core body temperature <35 °C. It can be classified as:

- Mild (>32–<35 °C)
- Moderate (30–32 °C)
- Severe (<30 °C)

(Resuscitation Council (UK), 2006)

Severe hypothermia is associated with a marked fall in cerebral blood flow and oxygen requirements, reduced cardiac output and decreased arterial pressure (Schneider, 1992). If there is rapid cooling prior to the development of hypoxaemia, decreased oxygen consumption and metabolism may precede the cardiac arrest and reduce organ ischaemia (Larach, 1995), exerting a protective effect on the brain and vital organs during cardiac arrest (Holzer *et al.*, 1997).

Core temperature-related cardiac arrhythmias can complicate hypothermia: sinus bradycardia, atrial fibrillation, VF and then finally asystole (Resuscitation Council (UK), 2006).

Table 9.1 Recognition and emergency treatment of calcium and magnesium disorders. Reproduced with permission of Resuscitation Council (UK).

Disorder	Causes	Presentation	ECG	Treatment
Hypercalcaemia Serum calcium concentration >2.6 mmol/l	Primary or tertiary hyperparathyroidism Malignancy Sarcoidosis Drugs	Confusion Weakness Abdominal pain Hypotension Arrhythmias Cardiac arrest	Short QT interval Prolonged QRS interval Flat T waves Atrioventricular (AV) block Cardiac arrest	Fluid replacement IV Furosemide 1 mg/kg IV Pamindronate 60–90 mg IV Calcitonin 4–8 units/kg/8 hours IM Review medication Haemodialysis
Hypocalcaemia Serum calcium concentration <2.1 mmol/l	Chronic renal failure Acute pancreatitis Calcium channel blocker overdose Toxic shock syndrome Rhabdomyolysis Tumour lysis syndrome	Paraesthesia Tetany Seizures AV block Cardiac arrest	Prolonged QT interval T wave inversion Heart block Cardiac arrest	Calcium chloride 10% 10–40 ml IV Magnesium sulphate 50% 4–8 mmol (if necessary) IV
Hypermagnesaemia Serum magnesium concentration >1.1 mmol/l	Renal failure Iatrogenic	Confusion Weakness Respiratory depression AV block Cardiac arrest	Prolonged PR and QT intervals T wave peaking AV block Cardiac arrest	Calcium chloride 10% 5–10 ml IV repeated if necessary Ventilatory support if necessary Saline diureses – 0.9% saline with furosemide 1 mg/kg IV Haemodialysis
Hypomagnesaemia Serum magnesium concentration <0.6 mmol/l	Gastrointestinal loss Polyuria Starvation Alcoholism Malabsorption	Tremor Ataxia Nystagmus Seizures Arrhythmias – torsade de pointes Cardiac arrest	Prolonged PR and QT intervals ST segment depression T wave inversion Flattened P waves Increased QRS duration Torsade de pointes	Severe or symptomatic: 2 g 50% magnesium sulphate (4 ml; 8 mmol) IV over 15 minutes Torsade de pointes: m2g 50% magnesium sulphate (4 ml; 8 mmol) IV over 1–2 minutes Seizure: 2 g 50% magnesium sulphate (4 ml; 8 mmol) IV over 10 minutes

If core temperature <30 °C, defibrillation is unlikely to be effective until rewarming is accomplished (Southwick & Dalglish, 1980). In the presence of hypothermia, the heart may not respond to cardioactive drugs and pacemaker stimulation (Reuler, 1978). Metabolism of drugs is reduced; following repeated administration, drugs can rise to toxic levels (Resuscitation Council (UK), 2006).

Death should not be confirmed until the patient has been rewarmed or until efforts to raise the core temperature have failed (Resuscitation Council (UK), 2006). Prolonged CPR may be required.

Cardiopulmonary resuscitation

All the principles of BLS and ALS apply to the hypothermic patient (Resuscitation Council (UK), 2006). However some modifications to the approach are required:

- Palpate a major artery, look for signs of life and observe the ECG monitor (if available) for up to 1 minute before diagnosing cardiac arrest (Resuscitation Council (UK), 2006); if a Dopplar probe is available, this can be used to determine whether there is peripheral blood flow (Soar *et al.*, 2005). Start chest compressions immediately if cardiac arrest is confirmed or if unsure whether a pulse is present or not
- Ventilate with warmed (40–46 °C) and humidified oxygen and consider careful tracheal intubation (Resuscitation Council (UK), 2006)
- Once CPR has started, confirm hypothermia using a low-reading thermometer; the same method for temperature measurement should be used throughout the resuscitation attempt to facilitate serial comparison of temperature readings (Resuscitation Council (UK), 2006); suggested methods for core temperature measurement include oesophageal, bladder, rectal and tympanic (Robinson *et al.*, 1998; Lefrant *et al.*, 2003)
- Prevent further heat loss if possible, e.g. remove wet clothing, cover the patient with a blanket
- In shock refractory VF/ventricular tachycardia (VT) (first three shocks are unsuccessful), defer further defibrillation attempts until core temperature >30 °C (Resuscitation Council (UK), 2006)

- Cannulate a central or large proximal vein
- Withhold drugs until the core temperature >30 °C; then double the standard time intervals between drug administration and use the lowest recommended drugs doses (Soar *et al.*, 2005); follow standard drug protocols once the core temperature returns towards normal (Resuscitation Council (UK), 2006)
- Handle the patient carefully – rough movement can precipitate cardiac arrhythmias

Rewarming

Although passive rewarming methods, e.g. warm blankets, warm environment, may suffice in cases of mild hypothermia (Kelly *et al.*, 2001), they will be ineffective if the patient is in cardiac arrest (Larach, 1995). In this situation active and rapid rewarming is essential (Carson, 1999). Core temperature rewarming methods include:

- Administration of warmed, humidified oxygen (40–46 °C)
- Infusion of warmed intravenous fluids
- Peritoneal, pleural or gastric lavage with warmed (40 °C) fluids
- Extracorpeal blood warming – this is the preferred method because it ensures adequate support of oxygenation and ventilation while the core body temperature is gradually rewarmed (Soar *et al.*, 2005; Resuscitation Council (UK), 2006)

The process of rewarming can cause vasodilation and an expansion of vascular space. Large volumes of fluids may need to be administered. In addition, severe hyperkalaemia may develop and will need correcting. Care should be taken to avoid hyperthermia.

Drowning

Drowning is defined as a process resulting in primary respiratory impairment from submersion/immersion in a liquid medium, i.e. a liquid–air interface is present at the entrance of the person's airway preventing him from breathing air (Idris *et al.*, 2003; Soar *et al.*, 2005).

Drowning is a common cause of accidental death in Europe, particularly in young males (Peden & McGee, 2003). In the UK in 2002, there were 427 deaths caused by drowning (Royal Society for the Prevention of Accidents, 2002). The consumption of alcohol is a contributory factor in up to 70% of drownings (Driscoll *et al.*, 2004).

Although survival following a prolonged submersion and prolonged CPR is rare, successful CPR associated with full neurological recovery is still possible in these circumstances (Siebke *et al.*, 1975; Southwick & Dalglish, 1980). The longest accurately documented cases of survival are 40 minutes under water and 2 hours under snow (Harris, 2004). Table 9.2 details the essential factors concerning a drowning incident.

The most significant and detrimental consequence of submersion is hypoxia, the duration of which is a critical factor in determining the patient's outcome (Soar *et al.*, 2005). Oxygenation, ventilation and perfusion are therefore of paramount importance.

Clearing the airways of aspirated water is not necessary (Rosen *et al.*, 1995). Approximately 10–15% of patients develop intense

Table 9.2 Essential factors concerning a drowning incident. Reproduced from Harris, M. (2004) Near drowning. In: Colquhoun M *et al.* (Eds) *ABC of Resuscitation*, 4th Ed. BMJ Books. Reprinted with permission from Wiley-Blackwell.

Factor	Comments
Length of time submerged	Favourable outcome associated with submersion for less than 5 minutes
Quality of immediate resuscitation	Favourable outcome if heartbeat can be restored at once
Temperature of water	Favourable outcome associated with submersion in ice cold water ($<5\,°C$)
Shallow water	Consider fracture/dislocation of cervical spine
A buoyancy aid being used by the casualty	Likely to be profoundly hypothermic. Victim may not have aspirated water
Nature of the water (fresh or salt)	Ventilation/perfusion mismatch from freshwater inhalation more difficult to correct. Risk of infection from river water high. Consider leptospirosis

laryngeal spasm which protects the lungs from aspiration of water or gastric contents ('dry drowning') (Skinner & Vincent, 1997). Even if water is aspirated, it is likely to be only small amounts, and it is rapidly absorbed into the central circulation (Rosen *et al.*, 1995). Vomiting/regurgitation of gastric contents is common (Manolios & Mackie, 1988).

Cardiopulmonary resuscitation

All the principles of BLS and ALS apply when undertaking CPR on a patient following submersion (Resuscitation Council (UK), 2006). However some modifications to the approach are required:

- Immobilise the cervical spine injury only if there are signs of severe injury or if the history suggests a severe injury (ILCOR, 2005), e.g. diving, use of a waterslide, signs of trauma or signs of alcohol intoxication (Soar *et al.*, 2005); cervical spine injury is associated with 0.5% of drowning incidents (Watson *et al.*, 2001). Apply jaw thrust, rather than head tilt and chin lift, to open the airway and immobilise the patient's spine using a cervical collar and spinal board or equivalent (Resuscitation Council (UK), 2006). Care should be taken if using a cervical collar because, if poorly applied, it can lead to an obstructed airway in an unconscious patient (Dodd *et al.*, 1995)
- Consider tracheal intubation at an early stage to protect the airway; regurgitation of gastric contents is common
- Insert a nasogastric tube, empty and decompress the stomach
- Administer antibiotics if there are signs of infection (more likely following drowning in a river)

In addition the patient may be hypothermic. The problems associated with undertaking CPR in the presence of hypothermia, together with specific modifications to the standard BLS and ALS protocols including rewarming, have been discussed earlier in the chapter.

Acute severe asthma

Acute severe asthma attacks are normally reversible and related deaths should be considered avoidable (Resuscitation Council

(UK), 2006). They are ten times more common at night (Brenner *et al.*, 1999) and most asthma-related deaths occur outside hospital. National guidelines recommend aggressive treatment (oxygen, beta-2 (β_2) agonist (e.g. salbutamol), corticosteroids and aminophylline) of acute severe asthma to prevent deterioration to cardiac arrest (see Figure 9.1) (British Thoracic Society, 2008).

Causes of cardiac arrest associated with acute severe asthma include:

- Severe bronchospasm and mucous plugging (Molfino *et al.*, 1991)
- Hypoxia-related cardiac arrhythmias
- Tension pneumothorax

Cardiopulmonary resuscitation

All the principles of BLS and ALS apply to undertaking CPR in a patient suffering a cardiac arrest following an acute severe asthma attack (Resuscitation Council (UK), 2006). However some modifications to the approach are required:

- Intubate the trachea as soon as possible because high resistance in the airways can hinder ventilation; high ventilation pressures are usually required and gastric distension usually occurs during bag/valve/mask ventilation
- Ensure prolonged inspiratory and expiratory times (ten inflations per minute) – this should avoid dynamic hyperinflation of the lungs and trapping of gases; if this is suspected during CPR, compress the chest wall and/or provide a period of apnoea to attempt to relieve the gas trapping (Resuscitation Council (UK), 2006)
- If dynamic hyperventilation is present, as it increases thransthoracic impedance (Deakin *et al.*, 1998), consider higher defibrillaion energies if initial defibrillation attempts are unsuccessful (Soar *et al.*, 2005)

N.B. high airway pressures required for ventilation can cause a tension pneumothorax – clinical features include unilateral chest wall expansion, tracheal displacement to the opposite side and subcutaneous emphysema (Resuscitation Council (UK), 2006). Emergency treatment is to release air from the pleural

MANAGEMENT OF ACUTE ASTHMA IN ADULTS	
ASSESSMENT OF SEVERE ASTHMA	
B	Healthcare professionals must be aware that patients with severe asthma and one or more adverse psychosocial factors are at risk of death
☑	• Keep patients who have had near fatal asthma or brittle asthma under specialist supervision indefinitely • A respiratory specialist should follow up patients admitted with severe asthma for at least 1 year after the admission

INITIAL ASSESSMENT	
MODERATE EXACERBATION	**LIFE THREATENING**

MODERATE EXACERBATION	LIFE THREATENING
• Increasing symptoms • PEF > 50–75% best or predicted • No features of acute severe asthma	In a patient with severe asthma any one of: • PEF < 33% best or predicted • SpO_2 <92% • PaO_2 <8 kPa • Normal $PaCO_2$ (4.6–6.0 kPa) • Silent chest
ACUTE SEVERE	• Cyanosis • Feeble respiratory effort
Any one of: • PEF 33–50% best or predicted • Respiratory rate ≥25/min Heart rate ≥110/min • Inability to complete sentences in one breath	• Bradycardia, arrhythmia, hypotension • Exhaustion, confusion, coma
	NEAR FATAL
	Raised $PaCO_2$ and/or requiring mechanical ventilation with raised inflation pressures

Clinical features	Severe breathlessness (including too breathless to complete sentences in one breath), tachypnoea, tachycardia, silent chest, cyanosis or collapse *None of these singly or together is specific and their absence does not exclude a severe attack*
PEF or FEV_1	PEF or FEV_1 are useful and valid measures of airway calibre. PEF expressed as a % of the patient's previous best value is most useful clinically. In the absence of this, PEF as a % of predicted is a rough guide
Pulse oximetry	Oxygen saturation (SpO_2) measured by pulse oximetry determines the adequacy of oxygen therapy and the need for arterial blood gas (ABG). The aim of oxygen therapy is to maintain SpO_2 ≥92%
Blood gases (ABG)	Patients with SpO_2 <92% or other features of life-threatening asthma require ABG measurement
Chest Radiography	Chest Radiography is not routinely recommended in the absence of: - suspected pneumomediastinum or pneumothorax - suspected consolidation - life-threatening asthma - failure to respond to treatment satisfactorily - requirement for ventilation

Fig. 9.1 BTS British Guidelines on the Management of Acute Asthma 2008. Courtesy of the BTS/SIGN Asthma Executive. (PEF: peak expiratory flow; FEV_1: forced expiratory volume in 1 second; PaO_2: arterial oxygen tension; $PaCO_2$: arterial blood carbon dioxide tension)

MANAGEMENT OF ACUTE ASTHMA IN ADULTS

CRITERIA FOR ADMISSION

B	Admit patients with any feature of a life-threatening or near fatal attack

B	Admit patients with any feature of a severe attack persisting after initial treatment

C	Patients whose peak flow is greater than 75% best or predicted 1 hour after initial treatment may be discharged from the emergency department, unless there are other reasons why admission may be appropriate

TREATMENT OF ACUTE ASTHMA

OXYGEN

C	• Give high flow oxygen to all patients with acute severe asthma
A	• In hospital, ambulance and primary care, nebulised β_2 agonist bronchodilators should be driven by oxygen
A	• Outside hospital, high-dose β_2 agonist bronchodilators may be delivered via large-volume spacers or nebulisers
C	• The absence of supplemental oxygen should not prevent nebulised therapy being given if indicated

β_2 AGONIST BRONCHODILATORS

A	Use high-dose inhaled β_2 agonist as first-line agents in acute asthma and administer as early as possible. Reserve intravenous β_2 agonist for those patients in whom inhaled therapy cannot be used reliably
☑	In acute asthma with life-threatening features the nebulised route (oxygen-driven) is recommended
A	In severe asthma (PEF or FEV_1 < 50% best or predicted) and asthma that is poorly responsive to an initial bolus dose of β_2 agonist, consider continuous nebulisation

STEROID THERAPY

A	Give steroids in adequate doses in all cases of acute asthma
☑	Continue prednisolone 40–50 mg daily for at least 5 days or unit recovery

IPRATROPIUM BROMIDE

B	Add nebulised ipratropium bromide (0.5 mg 4–6 hourly) to β_2 agonist treatment for patients with acute severe or life-threatening asthma or those with a poor initial response to β_2 agonist therapy

OTHER THERAPIES

B	Consider giving a single dose of IV magnesium sulphate for patients with: • Acute severe asthma who have not had a good initial response to inhaled bronchodilator therapy • Life-threatening or near fatal asthma
☑	IV magnesium sulphate (1.2-2 g IV infusion over 20 minutes) should only be used following consultation with senior medical staff
B	Routine prescription of antibiotics is not indicated for acute asthma

REFERRAL TO INTENSIVE CARE

Refer any patient:
• Requiring ventilatory support
• With acute severe or life threatening asthma, failing to respond to therapy, evidenced by:
 - deteriorating PEF
 - persisting or worsening hypoxial
 - hyercapnia
 - ABG analysis showing ↓ pH or ↑ H^+
 - exhaustion, feeble respiration
 - drowsiness, confusion
 - coma or respiratory arrest

Fig. 9.1 *Continued*

space with needle decompression, by inserting a large-gauge cannula in the second intercostal space, mid-clavicular line, taking care not to puncture the lung (Soar *et al.*, 2005).

Electrocution

Electrocution can result from domestic or industrial electricity, or from a lightning strike. Electrocution injuries in adults are mainly occur in the work environment and are associated with high voltage, while electrocution injurues in children mainly occur at home and are associated with low voltage (Soar *et al.*, 2005).

Lightning strike injuries have a mortality rate of 30% with 70% of those who survive sustaining significant morbidity (Stewart, 2000). Worldwide, lightning strikes cause 1000 deaths each year (Morbidity & Mortality Weekly Report, 1998). Injury can also occur indirectly through the ground from current splashing from a tree or similar object, which has been struck by lightning (Zafren *et al.*, 2005).

Factors effecting severity of the injury

Factors effecting the severity of electrical injury include magnitude of energy delivered, voltage, resistance to current flow, type of current, duration of contact with the source of the current and current pathway (Resuscitation Council (UK), 2006).

Skin resistance is the most important factor impeding the flow of current; it is reduced significantly by moisture, turning a minor injury into a life-threatening one (Wallace, 1991).

Types of current

There are two types of current:

- *Direct current (DC)*: present in batteries and lightning, the current flows in one direction for the duration of discharge. Induces one strong muscular contraction that often throws the casualty away from the current source (Fontanarosa, 1993). Asystole is more common after a DC shock (Soar *et al.*, 2005)
- *Alternating current (AC)*: present in most household and commercial sources of electricity. Contact with it may cause tetanic

skeletal muscle contractions, preventing self-release from the current source (Soar *et al.*, 2005). The repetitive frequency of AC increases the risk of current flow through the myocardium during the vulnerable refractory period of the cardiac cycle, which can cause VF (Geddes *et al.*, 1986)

Transthoracic current flow (hand-to-hand current pathway) is more likely to be fatal than a vertical current pathway (hand-to-foot) or a straddle current pathway (foot-to-foot) (Thompson & Ashwal, 1983).

Clinical effects on the patient

Electrocution injuries result from the direct effects of the current on cell membranes and vascular smooth muscle, and the production of heat energy as it passes through body tissues (American Heart Association (AHA) & International Liaison Committee on Resuscitation (ILCOR), 2000).

Cardiac arrest, VF or asystole, is the primary cause of death in patients following electrocution (Homma *et al.*, 1990). Respiratory arrest can be caused by a variety of different mechanisms:

• Passage of electric current through the brain inhibiting the respiratory centre in the medulla
• Tetanic contraction of the diaphragm and chest wall during exposure to the current
• Prolonged paralysis of the respiratory muscles
(AHA & ILCOR, 2000)

Electrical injuries often cause related trauma, e.g. cervical spine injury (Epperly & Stewart, 1989) and skin burns.

Cardiopulmonary resuscitation

All the principles of BLS and ALS apply to undertaking CPR in a patient suffering a cardiac arrest following electrocution (Resuscitation Council (UK), 2006). However some modifications to the approach are required:

• If applicable, ensure environment is safe and there is no electrocution risk to the team

- Immobilise the cervical spine and apply jaw thrust (rather than head tilt and chin lift) to open the airway
- Intubate early, particularly if there are burns to the face, mouth or neck (soft-tissue oedema may rapidly develop and obstruct the airway) (Resuscitation Council (UK), 2006)
- As muscular paralysis may persist for several hours following electrocution (Kleinschmidt-DeMasters, 1995), monitor breathing and provide assisted ventilation as required (Resuscitation Council (UK), 2006)
- Remove any smouldering clothes or shoes to prevent further thermal injury
- Administer sufficient fluids to maintain adequate diuresis to excrete by-products of tissue production including potassium and myoglobin (Cooper, 1995)
- Continue CPR for prolonged periods if required
- Request surgical expertise if there are severe thermal injuries

Pregnancy

Cardiac arrest in pregnancy is very rare, occurring in 1:30000 deliveries (Department of Health, 2004). Causes include haemorrhage, eclampsia, pulmonary embolism and amniotic fluid embolism (Jevon & Raby, 2001; Department of Health, 2004).

Anatomical and physiological changes in late pregnancy can make maternal CPR difficult. In particular, pressure by the gravid uterus on the major abdominal blood vessels can have profound effects on the circulation while the mother is in a supine position.

The main objective must be to prevent cardiopulmonary arrest. Assess the patient following the ABCDE approach (see Chapter 3). Key priorities include:

- Placing the mother in the left lateral position to relieve caval compression
- Administering 100% oxygen
- Administering a fluid bolus intravenously
- Seeking expert help early

(Jevon & Raby, 2001)

Cardiopulmonary resuscitation

All the principles of BLS and ALS apply to undertaking CPR in a patient suffering a cardiac arrest in pregnancy (Resuscitation Council (UK), 2006). However some modifications to the approach are required:

- Involve an obstetrician and a paediatrician at an early stage
- Position the mother in the left lateral tilt position at an angle of 15 degrees (Kinsella, 2003) – a wedge or similar can be used (Figure 9.2)
- Perform tracheal intubation (with correctly applied cricoid pressure) to protect the airway (there is a high risk of regurgitation of gastric contents); it is possible that a smaller tracheal tube than normal (0.5–1.0 mm internal diameter smaller than that usually used in a non-pregnant woman), will be required because oedema and swelling can narrow the mother's airway (Johnson *et al.*, 1998). In addition, as tracheal intubation in late pregnancy can be difficult (Rahman & Jenkins, 2005), senior anaesthetic help, a 'failed intubation drill' and alternative airway devices may be required (Henderson *et al.*, 2004)

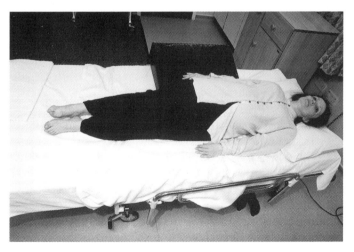

Fig. 9.2 Resuscitation in late pregnancy: position the mother in the left lateral tilt.

- Perform chest compressions slightly higher on the sternum; this is to adjust for the shifting of pelvic and abdominal contents towards the head
- Consider the use of abdominal ultrasound to identify the possible cause of the cardiac arrest (Soar *et al.*, 2005)
- Perform caesarean section if CPR is unsuccessful after 5 minutes; this will improve the chances of survival for both the mother and baby (Resuscitation Council (UK), 2006)

Poisoning

Poisoning is a leading cause of cardiac arrest in the <40 years age group (Watson *et al.*, 2004; Resuscitation Council (UK), 2006). Long-term survival following a cardiac arrest associated with poisoning is approximately 24% (AHA & ILCOR, 2000).

With some poisoning agents, cardiac arrest results from direct cardiotoxicity, while with others it is secondary to respiratory arrest caused by central nervous system (CNS) depression or aspiration of gastric contents. Pulseless electrical activity (PEA), a common complication of ingestion of drugs with negative inotropic properties, carries a far better prognosis in poisoning than when associated with a primary cardiac cause (Resuscitation Council (UK), 2000).

The emphasis is on intensive supportive therapy, correcting hypoxia, acid–base and electrolyte disorders (Resuscitation Council (UK), 2006).

Prevention of cardiac arrest

Prevention of cardiorespiratory arrest is a priority: follow the ABCDE approach to assess and treat the patient (Soar *et al.*, 2005), while waiting for the poison to be eliminated (Zimmerman, 2003). Particular attention to maintaining a clear airway and adequate breathing is required; a decreased level of consciousness can be associated with poisoning, which can lead to a compromised airway and inadequate ventilation, resulting in cardiorespiratory arrest and death (this is not uncommon) (Resuscitation Council (UK), 2006).

Specific therapeutic measures

As stated above, the emphasis is ongoing intensive supportive therapy, correcting hypoxia, acid–base and electrolyte disorders; very few therapeutic therapies are helpful (Resuscitation Council (UK), 2006). However, the following may be considered:

- *Activated charcoal*: although it can absorb certain drugs, its value decreases over time and there is no evidence that it improves survival (Soar *et al.*, 2005); a single dose of activated charcoal is recommended when a potential toxic amount of poison (which is known to be absorbed by activated charcoal) has been ingested <60 minutes previously (Chyka *et al.*, 2005); repeated doses may be helpful in life-threatening poisoning with carbemazepine, phenobarbital, quinine, theophylline and dapsone (Soar *et al.*, 2005). Activated charcoal must not be administered unless the patient can maintain his own airway or if the airway is secured with a tracheal tube
- *Gastric lavage*: this is only useful if the poison has been ingested <60 minutes previously and generally only following tracheal intubation (Soar *et al.*, 2005); delayed gastric lavage is not helpful and may in fact push the poison further down the gastrointestinal tract (Vale & Kulig, 2004)
- *Whole bowel irrigation*: this can be useful in some situations, e.g. potentially toxic ingestion of certain sustained-release or enteric medications and iron, removal of packets containing illicit drugs (Resuscitation Council (UK), 2006)
- *Haemodialysis*: this can be useful for eliminating life-threatening drugs or metabolites that are water soluble, have a low volume of distribution and low plasma protein bonding, e.g. methanol, salicylates (Golper & Bennett, 1988)
- *Specific antidotes*: e.g. N-acetylcysteine (paracetamol poisoning), naloxone (opiates) and flumazenil (benzodiazepines) (caution in patients who have benzodiazepine dependence or have co-ingested proconvulsant medication, e.g. tricyclic antidepressant, as significant toxicity may occur (Pitetti *et al.*, 2003)

Specific antidotes for poisons causing cardiorespiratory arrest

Opiates
Clinical features include respiratory depression, pin-point pupils and unconsciousness. Initially administer naloxone (narcan)

400 µg IV (Wanger *et al.*, 1998); repeated doses may be required because the duration of its action is approximately 45–70 minutes, whereas respiratory depression can perisist for up to 5 hours following opiate poisoning (Soar *et al.*, 2005). The prognosis is poor in patients with cardiac arrest secondary to opiate poisoning because it is usually preceded by respiratory depression/arrest, causing severe brain hypoxia (Sporer *et al.*, 1996). Naloxone can cause severe withdrawal symptoms, e.g. agitation, ventricular arrhythmias and pulmonary oedema, in patients with opiate dependence; in these patients, it should be used with caution (Resuscitation Council (UK), 2006).

Tricyclic anti-depressants
Tricyclic anti-depressants can lead to convulsions, hypotension and cardiac arrhythmias (British Medical Association & Royal Pharmaceutical Society of Great Britain, 2008). Most life-threatening complications occur within 6 hours of ingestion (Resuscitation Council (UK), 2006). Sodium bicarbonate reduces the toxicity (Sasyniuk *et al.*, 1986). Administration of hypertonic saline may be effective at treating cardiac toxicity (Brogan *et al.*, 1991).

Cocaine toxicity
Cocaine toxicity causes excess stimulation of the sympathetic nervous system, which may cause agitation, tachycardia, hypertensive crisis, hyperthermia and coronary vasoconstriction (Resuscitation Council (UK), 2006). Small doses of an intravenous benzodiazepine, e.g. midazolam, are effective as a first-line therapy (Soar *et al.*, 2005); glyceryl trinitrate can be effective at treating cocaine-induced vasoconstriction (McKinney & Rasmussen, 2003), but is only recommended as second-line therapy (Resuscitation Council (UK), 2006).

Cardiopulmonary resuscitation

All the principles of BLS and ALS apply to undertaking CPR in a patient suffering a cardiac arrest following poisoning (Resuscitation Council (UK), 2006). However some modifications to the approach are required:

- If necessary, ensure relevant precautions are taken if the poisoning is due to gas, corrosives etc.

- Intubate the patient as soon as possible, as there is a high incidence of pulmonary aspiration of gastric contents associated with poisoning
- If possible identify the poison(s) ingested: information from the patient's relatives and friends and ambulance crew may be of help. Also examine the patient for needle puncture marks, tablet bottles/sachets, odours, and corrosion around the mouth
- Access TOXBASE or telephone the National Poisons Information Service if specialist help and advice are required
- Continue CPR for prolonged periods if required, as the poison may be metabolised or excreted during this time (Resuscitation Council (UK), 2006)

Trauma

Cardiac arrest associated with blunt trauma has a poor prognosis (Rosemurgy *et al.*, 1993). Cardiac arrest associated with penetrating trauma has a marginally better prognosis (Bickell *et al.*, 1994). Overall, survival rates are 2.2%; a significant number of these patients have neurological disability (Resuscitation Council (UK), 2006).

Causes of cardiac arrest in a trauma patient include hypoxia, tension pneumothorax, hypovolaemia and cardiac tamponade (Resuscitation Council (UK), 2006).

Prevention of cardiorespiratory arrest

The patient should be assessed and treated following the ABCDE approach. While ensuring cervical spine immobilisation, ensure the patient has a patent airway, adequate breathing and adequate circulation; treat any life-threatening problems, e.g. tension pneumothorax, severe haemorrhage, and involve senior help, e.g. surgeon, at an early stage.

Cardiopulmonary resuscitation

All the principles of BLS and ALS apply to undertaking CPR in a patient suffering a cardiac arrest following trauma (Resuscitation Council (UK), 2006). However some modifications to the approach are required:

- Perform jaw thrust, not head tilt and chin lift, to open the airway
- Immobilise the cervical spine
- Exclude tension pneumothorax when ventilating
- Site two wide-bore cannulae and administer volume replacement if indicated
- Request surgical expertise and treat any life-threatening problems

Cardiovascular collapse or cardiac arrest caused by local anaesthetic

The administration of large doses of local anaesthetic (e.g. in operating rooms, labour wards, emergency department, radiology suite) can cause cardiac arrest (Resuscitation Council (UK), 2008). Twenty percent lipid emulsion has been shown to be effective to treat local anaesthetic induced cardiovascular collapse (Foxall *et al.*, 2007), cardiac arrhythmias (Ludot *et al.*, 2008) and cardiac arrest (Litz *et al.*, 2006, Rosenblatt *et al.*, 2006; Warren *et al.*, 2008).

The Resuscitation Council (UK) has issued guidance on cardiac arrest or cardiovascular collapse caused by local anaesthetic (Resuscitation Council (UK), 2008). This is based on other previously issued guidance (Picard & Meek, 2006; Association of Anaesthetists of Great Britain and Ireland, 2007). In addition, it is recommended that 500–1000 ml 20% lipid emulsion is immediately available for the treatment of severe cardiovascular compromise or cardiac arrest associated with local anaesthetic toxicity in all clinical areas where high doses of local anaesthetics are administered (Resuscitation Council (UK), 2008).

Prevention of cardiorespiratory arrest

The patient should be assessed following the ABCDE approach. If there is severe cardiovascular compromise (hypotension, unstable arrhythmias) that is attributable to local anaesthetic toxicity, begin treatment with 20% lipid emulsion 1.5 ml/kg (100 ml in 70 kg patient) IV as this may prevent cardiac arrest (Resuscitation Council (UK), 2008).

Cardiopulmonary resuscitation

All the principles of BLS and ALS apply to undertaking CPR in a patient who develops a cardiac arrest that is likely to have been caused by local anaesthetic toxicity. However, some modifications to the approach are required:

- Administer 20% lipid emulsion 1.5 ml/kg (100 ml in 70 kg patient) IV
- Commence an infusion of 20% lipid emulsion at 0.25 ml/kg/min (about 20 ml/min in 70 kg patient) and continue until a stable and adequate circulation has been restored (this may take up to 60 minutes to achieve)
- Repeat the above bolus dose every 5 minutes until the return of spontaneous circulation
- Report the case of suspected local anaesthetic intoxication to the National Patient Safety Agency (www.npsa.nhs.uk)

(Resuscitation Council (UK), 2008)

Chapter summary

Resuscitation in certain special situations requires modification to the standard BLS and ALS guidelines if the chances of survival are to be optimised. The special situations described in this chapter account for a large proportion of cardiac arrests in younger persons. As there is often no co-existing cardiorespiratory disease, prognosis is relatively good as long as effective CPR is instigated promptly. The key principles of CPR in these special situations have been discussed.

References

American Heart Association & International Liaison Committee on Resuscitation (2000) Guidelines 2000 for Cardiopulmonary Resuscitation and Emergency Cardiovascular Care – An international consensus on science. *Resuscitation* **46**:1–448.

Association of Anaesthetists of Great Britain and Ireland (2007) *Guidelines for the Management of Severe Local Anaesthetic Toxicity*. AAGBI, London, www.aagbi.org.

Bickell W, Wall Jr M, Pepe P *et al.* (1994) Immediate versus delayed fluid resuscitation for hypotensive patients with penetrating torso injuries. *New England Journal of Medicine* **331**:1105–9.

Bowden D (2001) Quoted from a lecture delivered by David Bowden, Former Consultant A & E, Manor Hospital, Walsall.

Brenner B, Chavda K, Karakurum M *et al.* (1999) Circadian differences among 4096 patients presenting to the emergency department with acute asthma. *Academic Emergency Medicine* **6**:523.

British Medical Association & Royal Pharmaceutical Society of Great Britain (2008) *BNF 55*. BMJ, London.

British Thoracic Society (2008) Management of Acute Asthma in Adults. British Thoracic Society, London.

Brogan W, Lange R, Kim A *et al.* (1991) Alleviation of cocaine-induced coronary vasoconstriction by nitroglycerin. *Journal of the American College of Cardiology* **18**:581–6.

Carson B (1999) Successful resuscitation of a 44 year old man with hypothermia. *Journal of Emergency Nursing* **25**(5):356–60.

Chyka P, Seger D, Krenzelok E, Vale J (2005) Position paper: single-dose activated charcoal *Clinical Toxicology* **43**:61–87.

Cohn J, Kowey P, Whelton P, Prisant L (2000) New guidelines for potassium replacement in clinical practice: a contemporary review by the National Council on Potassium in Clinical Practice. *Archives of Internal Medicine* **160**:2429–36.

Cooper M (1995) Emergent care of lightening and electrical injuries. *Seminars in Neurology* **15**:268–78.

Deakin C, McLarren R, Petley G *et al.* (1998) Effects of positive end-expiratory pressure on transthoracic impedance – implications for defibrillation. *Resuscitation* **37**:9–12.

Department of Health (2004) *Why Mothers Die. Report on the Confidential Enquires into Maternal Deaths in the United Kingdom 2000–2002*. The Stationery Office, London.

Dodd F, Simon E, McKeown D, Patrick M (1995) The effect of a cervical collar on the tidal volume of anaesthetised adult patients. *Anaesthesia* **50**:961–3.

Driscoll T, Harrison J, Steenkamp M (2004) Review of the role of alcohol in drowning associated with recreational aquatic activity. *Injury Prevention* **10**:107–13.

Epperly T, Stewart J (1989) The physical effects of lightening injury. *Journal of Family Practice* **29**:267–72.

Fontanarosa P (1993) Electric shock and lightening strike. *Annals of Emergency Medicine* **22**(2):378–87.

Foxall G, McCahon R, Lamb J, Hardman J, Bedforth N (2007) Levobupivacaine-induced seizures and cardiovascular collapse treated with Intralipid®. *Anaesthesia* **62**:516–8.

Geddes L, Bourland J, Ford G (1986) The mechanism underlying sudden death from electric shock. *Medical Instrumentation* **20**:303–15.

Golper T, Bennett W (1988) Drug removal by continuous arteriovenous haemofiltration. *Medical Toxicology and Adverse Drug Experience* **3**:341.

Harris M (2004) Near drowning. In: Colquhoun M *et al.* (eds) *ABC of Resuscitation*, 5th Ed. BMJ Books, London.

Henderson J, Popat M, Latto I, Pearce A (2004) Difficult airway society guidelines for management of the unanticipated difficult intubation. *Anaesthesia* **59**:675–94.

Holzer M, Behringer W, Schorkhuber W *et al.* (1997) Hypothermia for Cardiac Arrest (HACA) Study Group, Mild hypothermia and outcome after CPR. *Acta Anaesthesiologica Scandinavica Suppl* **111**:55–8.

Homma S, Gillam L, Weyman A (1990) Echocardiographic observations in survivors of acute electrical injury. *Chest* **97**:103–5.

Idris A, Berg R, Bierens J *et al.* (2003) Recommended guidelines for uniform reporting of data from drowning: The Utstein style. *Resuscitation* **59**:45–57.

International Liaison Committee on Resuscitation 2005 (2005) International consensus on cardiopulmonary resuscitation and emergency cardiovascular care science and treatment recommendations. *Resuscitation* **67**:157–341.

Jevon P, Raby M (2001) *Resuscitation in Pregnancy*. Butterworth Heinemann, Oxford.

Johnson M, Luppi C, Over D (1998) Cardiopulmonary resuscitation. In: Gambling D, Douglas M (Eds) *Obstetric Anaesthesia and Uncommon Disorders*. WB Saunders, Philadephia.

Kelly M, Ewens B, Jevon P (2001) Hyopthermia management. *Nursing Times* **97**(9):36–7.

Kinsella S (2003) Lateral tilt for pregnant women: why 15 degrees? *Anaesthesia* **58**:835–6.

Kleinschmidt-DeMasters B (1995) Neuropathology of lightening strike injuries. *Seminars in Neurology* **15**:323–8.

Larach M (1995) Accidental hypothermia. *Lancet* **345**:493–8.

Lefrant J, Muller L, de La Coussaye J *et al.* (2003) Temperature measurement in intensive care patients: comparison of urinary bladder, oesophageal, rectal, axillary and inguinal methods versus pulmonary artery core method. *Intensive Care Medicine* **29**:414–8.

Litz R, Popp M, Stehr S, Koch T (2006) Successful resuscitation of a patient with ropivacaine-induced asystole after axillary plexus block using lipid infusion. *Anaesthesia* **61**:800–1.

Ludot H, Tharin J, Belouadah M, Mazoit J, Malinovsky J (2008) Successful resuscitation after ropivacaine and lidocaine-induced ventricular arrhythmia following posterior lumbar plexus block in a child. *Anesthesia & Analgesia* **106**:1572–4.

Manolios N, Mackie I (1988) Drowning and near drowning on Australian beaches patrolled by life-savers: a 10-year study 1973–1983. *Medical Journal of Australia* **148**:170–1.

McKinney P, Rasmussen R (2003) Reversal of severe tricylic antidepressant-induced cardiotoxicity with intravenous hypertonic saline solution. *Annals of Emergency Medicine* **42**:20–4.

Molfino N, Nannani A, Matelli A *et al.* (1991) Respiratory arrest in near fatal asthma. *New England Journal of Medicine* **99**:358–62.

Morbidity & Mortality Weekly Report (1998) Lightening-associated deaths – United States 1980–1995. *MMWR Morbidity & Mortality Weekly Report* **47**:391–4.

Peden M, McGee K (2003) The epidemiology of drowning worldwide. *Injury Control & Safety Promotion* **10**:195–9.

Picard J, Meek T (2006) Lipid emulsion to treat overdose of local anaesthetic: the gift of the glob. *Anaesthesia* **61**:107–9.

Pitetti R, Singh S, Pierce M (2003) Safe and efficacious use of procedural sedation and analgesia by non-anesthesiologists in a pediatric emergency department. *Archives of Pediatrics & Adolescent Medicine* **157**:1090–6.

Rahman K, Jenkins J (2005) Failed tracheal intubation in obstetrics: no more frequent but still badly managed. *Anaesthesia* **60**:168–71.

Rastegar A, Soleimani M (2001) Hypokalaemia and hyperkalaemia. *Postgraduate Medical Journal* **77**:759–64.

Resuscitation Council (UK) (2006) *Advanced Life Support*, 5th Ed. Resuscitation Council (UK), London.

Resuscitation Council (UK) (2008) Cardiac arrest or cardiovascular collapse caused by local anaestheti. http://www.resus.org.uk/pages/caLocalA.htm. Accessed 5 April 2009.

Reuler J (1978) Hypothermia: pathophysiology, clinical settings and management. *Annals of Internal Medicine* **89**:519–27.

Robinson J, Charlton J, Seal R *et al.* (1998) Oesophageal, rectal, axillary, tympanic and pulmonary artery temperatures during cardiac surgery. *Canadian Journal of Anaesthesia* **45**:317–23.

Rosemurgy A, Norris P, Olson S *et al.* (1993) Prehospital traumatic cardiac arrest: the cost of futility. *Journal of Trauma* **35**:473–4.

Rosen P, Stoto M, Harley J (1995) The use of the Heimlich maneuver in near drowning: Institute of Medicine report. *Journal of Emergency Medicine* **13**:397–405.

Rosenblatt M, Abel M, Fischer G, Itzkovich C, Eisenkraft J (2006) Successful use of a 20% lipid emulsion to resuscitate a patient after a presumed bupivacaine-related cardiac arrest *Anesthesiology* **105**:217–8.

Royal Society for the Prevention of Accidents (2002) http://www.rospa.com/leisuresafety/water/statistics/stats_chart2001.pdf. Accessed 23 April 2009.

Sasyniuk BI, Jhamandas V, Valois M (1986) Experimental amitriptyline intoxication: treatment of cardiac toxicity with sodium bicarbonate. *Annals of Emergency Medicine* **15**(9):1052–9.

Siebke H, Rod T, Breivik H, Link B (1975) Survival after 40 minutes; submersion without cerebral sequelae. *Lancet* **1**:1275–7.

Skinner D, Vincent R (1997) *Cardiopulmonary Resuscitation*, 2nd Ed. Oxford University Press, Oxford.

Soar J, Deakin C, Nolan J *et al.* (2005) European Resuscitation Council Guidelines for Resuscitation 2005 Section 7. Cardiac arrest in special circumstances. *Resuscitation* **6751**:S135–70.

Southwick F, Dalglish Jr P (1980) Recovery after prolonged asystolic cardiac arrest in profound hypothermia: a case report and literature review. *Journal of the American Medical Association* **243**:1250–3.

Sporer K, Firestone J, Issacs S (1996) Out-of-hospital treatment of opoid overdoses in an urban setting. *Academic Emergency Medicine* **3**:660–7.

Stewart C (2000) When lightening strikes. *Emergency Medical Services* **29**(57–67):103.

Thompson J, Ashwal S (1983) Electrical injuries in children. *American Journal of Diseases of Children* **137**:231–5.

Vale J, Kulig K (2004) Position paper: gastric lavage. *Clinical Toxicology* **42**:933–43.

Wanger K, Brough L, Macmillan I *et al.* (1998) Intravenous vs. subcutaneous naloxone for out-of-hospital management of presumed opoid overdose. *Academic Emergency Medicine* **5**:293–9.

Wallace J (1991) Electrical injuries. In: *Harrison's Principles of Internal Medicine*, 12th Ed. McGraw-Hill, New York.

Warren J, Thoma R, Georgescu A, Shah S (2008) Intravenous lipid infusion in the successful resuscitation of local anesthetic-induced cardiovascular collapse after supraclavicular brachial plexus block. *Anesthesia & Analgesia* **106**:1578–80.

Watson R, Cummings P, Quan L *et al.* (2001) Cervical spine injuries among submersion victims. *Journal of Trauma* **51**:658–62.

Watson W, Litovitz T, Klein-Schwartz W *et al.* (2004) 2003 annual report of the American Association of Poison Control Centers Toxic Exposure Surveillance System. *American Journal of Emergency Medicine* **22**:335–404.

Wyatt J, Illingworth R, Clancy M *et al.* (2006) *Oxford Handbook of Accident & Emergency Medicine*, 2nd Ed. Oxford University Press, Oxford.

Zafren K, Durrer B, Herry J, Brugger H (2005) Lightning injuries: prevention and on-site treatment in mountains and remote areas. Official guidelines of the International Commission for Mountain Emergency Medicine and the Medical Commission of the International Mountaineering and Climbing Federation (ICAR and UIAA MEDCOM). *Resuscitation* **65**:369–72.

Zimmerman J (2003) Poisonings and overdoses in the intensive care unit: general and specific management issues. *Critical Care Medicine* **31**:2794.

Chapter 10

Anaphylaxis

Introduction

Anaphylaxis is an acute, severe, hypersensitivity reaction that can lead to asphyxia, cardiovascular collapse and cardiac arrest. The incidence is on the increase (Department of Health, 2006), probably associated with a notable increase in the prevalence of allergic diseases in the last 30 years (Working Group of the Resuscitation Council (UK), 2008). It is often poorly managed; in particular, adrenaline is greatly under-used.

In 2008, The Resuscitation Council (UK) published its revised guidelines on the emergency treatment (Working Group of the Resuscitation Council (UK), 2008).

The aim of this chapter is to understand the emergency treatment of anaphylaxis.

Learning outcomes

At the end of the chapter the reader will be able to:

- Provide a definition of anaphylaxis
- Discuss the incidence of anaphylaxis
- Discuss the pathophysiology of anaphylaxis
- List the causes of anaphylaxis
- Describe the clinical features and diagnosis of anaphylaxis
- Discuss the treatment of anaphylaxis

Definition

Anaphylaxis can be defined as 'a severe, life-threatening, generalised or systemic hypersensitivity reaction' (Johansson *et al.*,

2004). Basically, it is a life-threatening allergic reaction – the extreme end of the allergic spectrum (Anaphylaxis Campaign, 2007).

The term anaphylactoid reaction was previously used to describe a severe allergic reaction that was not IgE mediated; causes include aspirin, exercise and blood products. It is clinically indistinguishable from an anaphylaxis reaction (Jevon, 2004) and the term is no longer used (Resuscitation Council (UK), 2006).

Incidence

The incidence of anaphylaxis is on the increase (Gupta *et al.*, 2007), probably associated with a notable increase in the prevalence of allergic diseases in the last 30 years (Working Group of the Resuscitation Council (UK), 2008). A review of the literature on the incidence of anaphylaxis shows that:

- The incidence of anaphylaxis in the general population has increased
- Since 1990, admissions for anaphylaxis have increased by 700% (Gupta *et al.*, 2007)
- In England, between 1990–91 and 2000–01, there were 13 230 admissions to hospital for anaphylaxis (Gupta *et al.*, 2003)
- Between 1991 and 1994 the number of discharges from hospitals in England with a diagnosis of anaphylaxis doubled from 415 to 876 (Sheikh & Alves, 2000)
- In 2004, 3171 patients were admitted to hospital with anaphylaxis in the UK (Peng & Jick, 2004)
- Anaphylaxis is more common in females than in males: in 2004, 58% of attendees to emergency departments with anaphylaxis were female, 42% were male (Peng & Jick, 2004). The findings of Webb & Lieberman (2006) were comparable: females (62%) and males (38%)
- The mean age of patient with anaphylaxis is 37 years (Webb & Lieberman, 2006)
- Approximately 1 in 3500 emergency department attendances are due to anaphylaxis (Stewart & Ewan, 1996)
- 50% of all anaphylactic reactions in the community are treated in the hospital, with 20% requiring admission (Uguz *et al.*, 2005)

- Death from anaphylaxis is becoming more common, particularly in children and young adults (Ewan, 2000).

(Jevon, 2008)

Pathophysiology

Irrespective of the mechanism of anphylaxis, mast cells and basophils release histamines and other vasoactive mediators, which produce circulatory, respiratory, gastrointestinal and cutaneous effects (Wyatt *et al.*, 2006). These effects can include the development of pharyngeal and laryngeal oedema, bronchospasm, decreased vascular tone and capillary leak causing circulatory collapse (Jevon, 2004).

Causes

Causes of anaphylaxis include:

- Drugs, e.g. penicillin, aspirin, anaesthetics
- Bee/wasp stings
- Foods, e.g. peanuts, tomatoes, fish
- Blood products
- Immunisations
- Latex
- Contrast media
- Drugs, e.g. antibiotics, aspirin

(Anaphylaxis Campaign, 2007; BNF, 2007)

In approximately 40% of anaphylactic reactions, the cause is unknown (idiopathic anaphylaxis) (Webb & Lieberman, 2006; Greenberger, 2007).

Clinical features and diagnosis

The lack of a consistent clinical picture can sometimes make an accurate diagnosis difficult (Project Team of the Resuscitation Council (UK), 2005). Anaphylaxis can vary in severity and the process can be slow, rapid or biphasic. A detailed history and examination are essential as soon as possible. The clinical presentation often includes:

- Urticaria
- Angioedema
- Respiratory distress
- Wheeze/stridor
- Cardiovascular shock
- Tachycardia and hypotension
- Pallor

(Jevon, 2004; Anaphylaxis Campaign, 2007)

Anaphylaxis can vary in severity and the onset is usually rapid, occasionally it may be delayed by a few hours and even persist for longer than 24 hours (Fisher, 1986). The patient feels unwell, usually has skin changes, e.g. urticaria and angioedema, and will have a compromised airway and/or breathing and/or circulation (Jevon, 2008). Death from anaphylaxis usually occurs within 10–15 minutes, with cardiovascular collapse the commonest cause of death (Resuscitation Council (UK), 2006).

It is possible to mistake a panic attack or a vasovagal attack for anaphylaxis and adrenaline has been administered inappropriately in these situations (Johnston *et al.*, 2003). The clinical features for both these presentations are as follows:

- *A panic attack*: hyperventilation, tachycardia and anxiety-related erythematous rash, but no hypotension, pallor, wheeze or urticarial rash
- *A vasovagal attack*: the absence of a rash, tachycardia and dyspnoea should rule out anaphylaxis as the cause of the collapse

(Jevon, 2006)

Measurement of mast cell tryptase levels is the specific test to confirm the diagnosis of anaphylaxis:

- *Minimum*: one sample 1–2 hours after the start of symptoms
- *Ideal*: three timed samples – as soon as feasibly possible after the start of the symptoms, 1–2 hours after the start of the

symptoms and 24 hours later (or in the allergy clinic); serial samples are preferable (Brown *et al.*, 2004)

(Working Group of the Resuscitation Council (UK), 2008)

Treatment of anaphylaxis

The Resuscitation Council (UK) algorithm for the treatment of anaphylaxis in adults is detailed in Figure 10.1. The treatment of anaphylaxis is as follows:

1. Assess the patient following the ABCDE approach described in Chapter 3
2. Request senior help
3. If able, stop or remove the probable cause of the anaphylaxis, e.g. if a blood transfusion is in progress, stop it
4. Recline the patient into a position of comfort and raise the legs (this position may be helpful in hypotension but unhelpful in respiratory distress)
5. Ensure the patient has a clear airway; if stridor is present, alert senior expert help immediately (in anaphylaxis, stridor is probably due to potentially life-threatening laryngeal oedema)
6. Administer high-flow oxygen (15 l/minute) using a non-rebreathe mask. Establish oxygen saturation monitoring using a pulse oximeter
7. Administer adrenaline 500 μg IM if indicated (see Figure 10.1)
8. Insert a wide-bore intravenous cannula (e.g. 14 gauge) and commence intravenous fluids: 1000 ml of 0.9% normal saline in the first hour, followed by 500 ml/hour in the next 2–3 hours (Wyatt *et al.*, 2006)
9. Establish continuous electrocardiogram (ECG) monitoring: cardiac arrhythmias can sometimes occur (Resuscitation Council (UK), 2006)
10. Closely monitor the patient's vital signs
11. Assess and reassess the patient following the ABCDE approach
12. Repeat the adrenaline after 5 minutes if there is no improvement

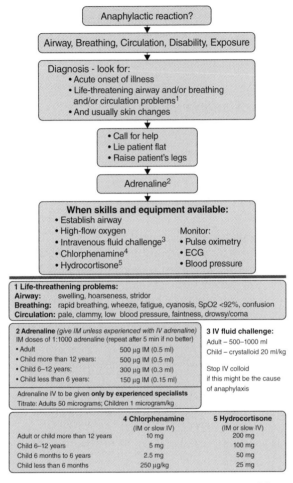

Fig. 10.1 Anaphylaxis algorithm. Reproduced with permission of Resuscitation Council (UK).

13. Do not sit the patient up or stand him up if he is feeling faint or dizzy – he may be in profound shock and may then have a cardiac arrest

(Working Group of the Resuscitation Council (UK), 2008)

Adrenaline

Adrenaline is the most important drug in anaphylaxis (Fisher, 1995). To be effective, it needs to be administered promptly (Patel *et al.*, 1994). Adrenaline:

- Reverses peripheral vasodilation
- Reduces oedema
- Dilates the airways
- Increases myocardial contractility
- Suppresses histamine and leukotriene release

The recommended dose of adrenaline is 500 μg IM (0.5 ml of 1:1000 solution) (Resuscitation Council (UK), 2008). This can be repeated after 5 minutes if there is no clinical improvement (Resuscitation Council (UK), 2008); several doses may be required (BNF, 2007). The intramuscular route is generally used for the administration of adrenaline as it is relatively safe and adverse effects are rare. The only reported severe adverse effect following intramuscular administration of adrenaline was a myocardial infarction in a patient with severe ischaemic heart disease (Saff *et al.*, 1993).

Cautions include the following:

- Two strengths of adrenaline are available: 1:1000 solution is used for intramuscular injection, while the 1:10000 solution is used for intravenous injection (Jevon, 2008)
- The subcutaneous route should not be utilised for the administration of adrenaline because absorption is considerably slower (Resuscitation Council (UK), 2008)

The more hazardous intravenous route is occasionally used, particularly if the patient is in profound shock which is judged to be immediately life threatening or in certain situations, e.g. anaesthesia (Resuscitation Council (UK), 2005). However, adrenaline administered intravenously can cause life-threatening cardiac arrhythmias, hypertension and myocardial ischaemia and is for specialist use only, e.g. anaesthetists, emergency physicians and intensive care doctors (Working Group of the Resuscitation Council (UK), 2008). It is recommended to titrate intravenous adrenaline using 50 μg (0.5 ml of 1:10000 solution) boluses; if repeated doses are required, an adrenaline infusion should be started (Working Group of the Resuscitation Council (UK), 2008). The patient should be on a cardiac monitor and resuscitation equipment should be immediately available.

Antihistamine

An antihistamine, e.g. chlorpheniramine (piriton), should be used routinely in anaphylaxis, though care should be taken to avoid drug-induced hypotension (BNF, 2007). The recommended dose is 10 mg either intramuscularly or by slow intravenous injection (Working Group of the Resuscitation Council (UK), 2008).

Hydrocortisone

Hydrocortisone should be administered following severe anaphylaxis to help prevent late sequelae, particularly in asthmatics who have been on corticosteroid treatment previously (Resuscitation Council (UK), 2005). The recommended dose is 200 mg either intramuscularly or by slow intravenous injection and care should be taken to avoid inducing further hypotension (Working Group of the Resuscitation Council (UK), 2008).

Intravenous fluids

If severe hypotension is present, a fluid challenge is recommended: 500–1000 ml of a crystalloid solution, e.g. 0.9% of normal saline, is suitable. Further infusion may be required (Working Group of the Resuscitation Council (UK), 2008).

Inhaled beta-2 agonist

Consider further bronchodilatory therapy, e.g. salbutamol (inhaled or intravenously) (Working Group of the Resuscitation Council (UK), 2008).

Cardiac arrest following anaphylaxis

All the principles of BLS and ALS apply to a patient with an anaphylaxis-induced cardiac arrest (Resuscitation Council (UK), 2006). In particular:

- Secure the airway with a tracheal tube as soon as possible – senior anaesthetic help will undoubtedly be required, particularly if laryngeal and/or pharyngeal oedema is present
- Administer adrenaline intravenously not intramuscularly
- Provide aggressive fluid resuscitation if shock was present prior to collapse

Follow up

Even if the reaction is only moderate, the patient should be warned of the possibility of an early recurrence of symptoms. Sometimes monitoring for 8–24 hours will be required, particularly when the reaction:

- Is severe and is of slow onset due to idiopathic anaphylaxis
- Occurs in a severe asthmatic
- Is complicated by a severe asthmatic attack
- Could be triggered again because further absorption of the allergen is possible

(Jevon, 2004)

Chapter summary

Anaphylaxis can be life threatening. This chapter has detailed the guidelines issued by the Resuscitation Council (UK) to treat it (Working Group of the Resuscitation Council (UK), 2008). Early treatment with intramuscular adrenaline is paramount.

References

Anaphylaxis Campaign (2007) www.anaphylaxis.org.uk. Accessed 8 September 2007.

Department of Health (2006) *A Review of Services for Allergy. The Epidemiology, Demand for, and Provision of Treatment and Effectiveness of Clinical Interventions.* Department of Health, London.

Ewan P (2000) *Anaphylaxis.* In: Durham S (Ed) *ABC of Allergies.* BMJ Books, London.

Fisher M (1986) Clinical observations on the pathophysiology and treatment of anaphylactic cardiovascular collapse. *Anaesthesia & Intensive Care* **14**:17–21.

Fisher M (1995) Treatment of acute anaphylaxis. *British Medical Journal* **311**:731–3.

Greenberger P (2007) Idiopathic anaphylaxis. *Immunology and Allergy Clinics of North America* **27**(2):273–93.

Gupta R, Sheikh A, Strachan D, Anderson H (2003) Increasing hospital admissions for systemic allergic disorders in England: an analysis of national admissions data. *British Medical Journal* **327**:1142–3.

Gupta R, Sheikh A, Strachan D, Anderson H (2007) Time trends in allergic disorders in the UK. *Thorax* **62**:91–6.

Jevon P (2004) *Anaphylaxis: A Practical Guide*. Butterworth Heinemann, Oxford.

Jevon P (2006) An overview of managing anaphylaxis in the community. *Nursing Times* **102**(39):48.

Jevon P (2008) Severe allergic reaction: management of anaphylaxis in hospital. *British Journal of Nursing* **17**(2):104–8.

Johansson S, Bieber T, Dhal R *et al.* (2004) Revised nomenclature for allergy for global use: Report of the Nomenclature review Committee of the World. *Journal of Allergy and Clinical Immunology* **113**(5):832–6.

Johnston S, Unsworth J, Gompels M (2003) Adrenaline given outside the context of life-threatening allergic reactions. *British Medical Journal* **326**(7389):589–90.

Patel L, Radivan FS, David TJ (1994) Management of anaphylactic reactions to food. *Archives of Disease in Childhood* **71**:370–5.

Peng M, Jick H (2004) A population based study of the incidence, cause and severity of anaphylaxis in the United Kingdom. *Archives of Internal Medicine* **164**(3):317–9.

Project Team of the Resuscitation Council (UK) (2005) *Emergency Medical Treatment of Anaphylactic Reactions*. Resuscitation Council (UK), London.

Resuscitation Council (UK) (2006) *Advanced Life Support*, 5th Ed. Resuscitation Council (UK), London.

Saff R, Nahhas A, Fink J (1993) Myocardial infarction induced by coronary vasospasm after self-administration of epinephrine. *Annals of Allergy* **70**:396–8.

Sheikh A, Alves B (2000) Hospital admissions for acute anaphylaxis: time trend study. *British Medical Journal* **320**:1441.

Stewart A, Ewan P (1996) The incidence, aetiology and management of anaphylaxis presenting to an accident & emergency department. *The Quarterly Journal of Medicine* **89**:859–64.

Uguz A, Lack G, Pumphrey R *et al.* (2005) Allergic reactions in the community: a questionnaire survey of members of the anaphylaxis campaign. *Clinical and Experimental Allergy* **35**(6):746–50.

Webb L, Lieberman P (2006) Anaphylaxis: a review of 601 cases. *Annals of Allergy, Asthma, & Immunology* **97**(1):39–43.

Working Group of the Resuscitation Council (UK) (2008) *Emergency Treatment of Anaphylactic Reactions: Guidelines for Healthcare Providers*. Resuscitation Council (UK), London.

Wyatt J, Illingworth R, Graham C *et al.* (2006) *Oxford Handbook of Emergency Medicine*, 3rd Ed. Oxford University Press, Oxford.

Chapter 11

Acute Coronary Syndromes

Rebecca McBride

Introduction

An acute myocardial infarction (AMI) can be classified as an ST segment elevation myocardial infarction (STEMI) or a non-ST segment elevation myocardial infarction (NSTEMI) and these, together with unstable angina, are recognised as part of a spectrum of clinical disease collectively referred to as acute coronary syndromes (ACS) (Resuscitation Council (UK), 2006).

Patients presenting with ACS require urgent assessment and investigations to confirm the diagnosis and establish the immediate risk of sudden cardiac death. The appropriate treatment should be commenced promptly and its effect evaluated.

The aim of this chapter is to understand the treatment of ACS.

Learning outcomes

At the end of the chapter the reader will be able to:

- Describe the pathogenesis of ACS
- Discuss the classification of ACS
- Outline the diagnosis of ACS
- Describe the immediate treatment of ACS
- Outline two methods of coronary reperfusion therapy

Pathogenesis of ACS

ACS is commonly caused by the rupture of an atheromatous plaque in a coronary artery (Chesebro *et al.*, 1997). Prior to rupture, most of these plaques are not haemodynamically significant

(Ambrose & Fuster, 1997). However once the plaque ruptures the following events are triggered:

- Haemorrhage into the plaque causing it to expand and restrict the lumen of the coronary artery
- Smooth muscle contraction of the artery wall, further restricting the lumen
- Thrombus formation on the surface of the ruptured plaque (platelet adhesion) leading to further constriction or even total obstruction of the coronary lumen

The degree and duration of occlusion, together with the presence or absence of collateral circulation, will determine the type of ACS that results (American Heart Association (AHA) & International Liaison Committee on Resuscitation (ILCOR), 2000).

Classification of ACS

Acute coronary syndromes can be classified as:

- Unstable angina
- Non-ST segment elevation myocardial infarction (NSTEMI)
- ST segment elevation myocardial infarction (STEMI)

Unstable angina

In unstable angina one or more of the following may be present:

- Crescendo angina – angina of effort occurring over a few days with increasing frequency and provoked by progressively less exertion
- Short episodes of angina, not specifically provoked by exertion, occurring recurrently and unpredictably
- Prolonged period of angina, not provoked by exertion, raising the suspicion of AMI but without electrocardiogram (ECG) and laboratory evidence

The ECG in a patient presenting with ACS may show ST segment depression reflecting myocardial ischemia, show non-specific abnormalities such as T wave inversion or in some instances be normal. Cardiac enzymes are usually normal and the troponin assay is either normal or very marginally raised (Resuscitation Council (UK), 2006).

Non ST segment elevation myocardial infarction

Patients present with the clinical features of an AMI accompanied by an ECG showing non-specific ECG abnormalities such as ST segment elevation or T wave inversion. Cardiac enzymes are elevated indicating that myocardial damage has occurred and a troponin assay is also raised.

ST segment elevation myocardial infarction

Patients present with the clinical features of an AMI accompanied by an ECG which shows the ST segment of some leads to be elevated, indicating myocardial damage; if left untreated, this results in Q waves forming in the leads reflecting the territory of the coronary artery affected by the fissuring of the atheromatous plaque. Cardiac enzymes will be raised and the troponin assay will reflect the myocardial damage.

Diagnosis of ACS

Clinical history

The presenting history of the patient is vital in establishing a diagnosis of ACS, particularly the timing of the onset of chest pain. Clinical features of ACS include:

- Central crushing chest pain, which may radiate down the left arm, into the back or neck or into the throat or jaw
- Nausea and vomiting
- Breathlessness
- Sweating and pallor

However, although it can help with diagnosis, the history can sometimes cause confusion. For example an ACS may develop without any significant chest pain, for example in the elderly, patients with diabetes and those in the peri-operative phase. Sometimes it is difficult to distinguish between cardiac and indigestion pain. Any severe pain can cause tachycardia, pallor, nausea and vomiting, all common clinical features of an ACS.

Nevertheless an accurate history does provide a baseline against which progress, deterioration and response to treatment can be detected (Resuscitation Council (UK), 2006).

Clinical examination

Clinical examination derives little benefit in establishing a diagnosis of ACS but may identify another cause for chest pain or identify other abnormalities, such as signs of heart failure or cardiac murmurs, which may influence investigations and treatment options. Clinical examination should provide a baseline against which changes due to the progression of the condition, patient deterioration or response to the ensuing treatment can be judged, (Resuscitation Council (UK), 2006). A systematic approach to examination should be adopted by professionals so that not only is the cardiovascular system examined, but also the respiratory and neurological systems, which can alter as a result of cardiovascular instability.

12-lead ECG

The 12-lead ECG is essential in the management of a patient with an ACS. It can help with diagnosis, provide a guide to the most appropriate treatment and, when repeated, can provide an indication to the progression of the ACS together with response to treatment.

The 12-lead ECG is also an essential element of risk assessment, both short and long term. For example, ST elevation or new left bundle branch block in a patient with a typical history of AMI is an indication for coronary reperfusion therapy. The presence of ST depression rather than elevation, however, would suggest that although coronary reperfusion therapy is unlikely to be beneficial in the short term, in the long term there is a high risk of further coronary events. These patients would undoubtedly benefit from further investigations and interventions.

The 12-lead ECG can also provide an indication to the site of myocardial damage and the coronary artery effected. This can also help predict prognosis, likely complications and sometimes the most appropriate treatment. The sites of AMI and their depiction on the 12-lead ECG are as follows:

- *Anterior or anteroseptal*: V1–V4 (usually left anterior descending coronary artery) (Figure 11.1)
- *Inferior*: II, III and aVF (usually right coronary artery, occasionally circumflex) (Figure 11.2)
- *Lateral*: V5–V6 and/or I and aVF (circumflex or diagonal branch of left anterior descending coronary artery) (Figure 11.3)
- *Posterior*: reciprocal changes (ST depression) together with dominant R waves in the anterior leads (usually right coronary artery, occasionally circumflex) (Figure 11.4)

Other ECGs can be performed which identify other regions of the heart subjected to myocardial damage, such as the right heart ECG. This is a mirror image of the standard chest leads, with all the limb leads remaining the same. The chest leads are then relabelled RV1 to RV6.

Another ECG that can be performed is that of the posterior surface of the myocardium where three electrodes are placed in the posterior region of the chest. These leads, labelled V7, V8 and V9, are placed in a horizontal line around the chest continuing from V6 where V7 is the posterior axillary line and V9 is to the left of the spine and V8 in the midline of those. It is important when performing additional ECGs that they are clearly labelled for interpretation purposes.

Laboratory investigations

Creatine kinase (CK), aspartate transaminase (AST) and lactate dehydrogenase (LDH) are enzymes released from damaged cardiac muscle; if elevated they may indicate cardiac damage. Unfortunately they are also released from skeletal muscle when it is damaged or during prolonged and vigorous exercise (Resuscitation Council (UK), 2006). The cardiospecific CK-MB can be measured, but is usually not routinely available.

Cardiac troponins (troponin 1 and troponin T) can also be measured, particularly as part of risk assessment. For example, if the troponin levels are raised 6–8 hours after the onset of pain in a patient with unstable angina, there is a greater risk of further

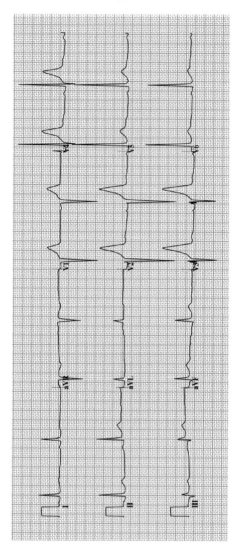

Fig. 11.1 Anterior myocardial infarction.

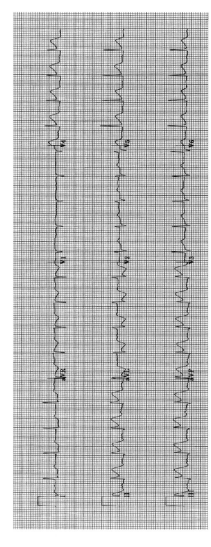

Fig. 11.2 Inferior myocardial infarction.

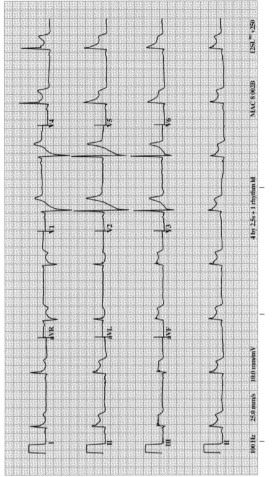

Fig. 11.3 Lateral myocardial infarction.

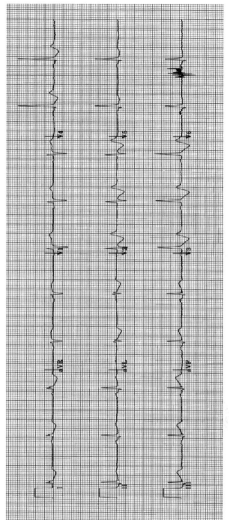

Fig. 11.4 Posterior myocardial infarction.

coronary events such as sudden death or a subsequent myocardial infarction than if the levels were normal (Resuscitation Council (UK), 2006). It is worth remembering that other conditions may release cardiac troponins since they are components of the contractile structure of myocardial cells, e.g. myocarditis, cardiac failure, sustained tachyarrhythmia, pulmonary embolism, acute sepsis and renal failure (Resuscitation Council (UK), 2005).

Echocardiography

Echocardiography is a useful investigation in the assessment of the left ventricle and any impairment arising from ACS. It is used to identify regional wall motion and also to assess the valvular structures, and also identifies any complications as a result of ACS or AMI.

Immediate treatment of ACS

General treatment measures for ACS

The patient should be assessed as soon as possible so that the most appropriate treatment can be started. The general treatment measures for all ACS are:

- Oxygen (high concentration) can reduce ST elevation in patients with anterior myocardial infarction (Maroko *et al.*, 1975)
- Glyceryl trinitrate: sublingual tablets or spray
- Aspirin 300 mg crushed or chewed
- Morphine or diamorphine intravenously, titrated to avoid sedation and respiratory depression

(Resuscitation Council (UK), 2006)

The majority of patients with ACS will be more comfortable sitting up. The supine position for these patients can sometime provoke or worsen the pain. The use of anti-emetics should also be considered.

ACS is the commonest cause of sudden death in most adults (Burke *et al.* 1999). Therefore continuous ECG monitoring should be established quickly since a cardiac arrhythmia may ensue; where possible a baseline rhythm strip should be recorded. In addition, to continuous cardiac monitoring access to defibrillation is vital should pulseless ventricular tachyarrhythmias occur.

Unstable angina and NSTEMI

The two key objectives of treatment for patients with unstable angina or NSTEMI are:

- To prevent new thrombus formation by reducing platelet aggregation
- Reduce myocardial oxygen demand since the myocardial cells have a limited supply of oxygen and glucose

(Resuscitation Council (UK), 2006)

The treatments advocated are for preventing further thrombus formation are:

- 75 mg aspirin daily (unless they have a known allergy) (ISIS 2, 1988)
- Low molecular weight heparin (LMWH) in weight-related doses, e.g. 1 mg/kg twice daily subcutaneously
- Clopidogrel with a loading dose of 300 mg, then a daily dose of 75 mg once daily especially if they are referred for percutaneous coronary intervention (PCI)
- If the patient is deemed at high risk then glycoprotein IIb/IIIa inhibitor (tirofiban) is commenced, the dose being calculated proportionate to the patient's weight. It is effective at reducing adverse cardiac events such as AMI and death (Kong *et al.*, 1998)

To reduce oxygen demand of the myocardial cells the following treatments are available:

- Continuous intravenous or buccal administration of nitrates will usually provide some benefit if sublingual administration of nitrates fails to settle chest pain; there are also benefits the patient with signs of cardiac failure, since it has homodynamic effects such as vasodilation of the venous capacitance vessels and the coronary arteries. The blood pressure should be higher than 90 mmHg systolic, however, since the blood pressure may drop with the administration of nitrates

- If not contraindicated, beta-adrenoceptor blocking drugs will help to reduce myocardial oxygen demand, control angina and/or reduce infarct size (ISIS 1, 1986). There is a lower incidence of ventricular fibrillation and supraventricular tachyarrhythmias in patients treated early with beta blockers (ISIS 1, 1986)
- Diltiazem may also be beneficial if beta-adrenoceptors are contraindicated
- The use of angiotensin converting enzyme (ACE) inhibitors should be considered, especially if echocardiography shows left ventricular systolic impairment or heart failure; it has been shown to reduce mortality in patients with AMI

Acute myocardial infarction with ST segment elevation or new left bundle branch block

As well as the general measures identified above, patients with AMI with ST segment elevation or who have a new left bundle branch block on their ECG should be considered for coronary reperfusion therapy. The aim of this therapy is to restore the blood supply to myocardium that has not yet been irreversibly damaged.

There are two common methods for establishing coronary reperfusion:

- Thrombolytic therapy
- PCI

Thrombolytic therapy is profoundly time dependent and particularly effective when given within the first 3 hours after the onset of chest pain; patients presenting within 12 hours of the commencement of their symptoms derive short- and long-term benefits.

The benefits of thrombolytic therapy in the management of AMI are well known. A recent overview of all randomised trials showed a short-term reduction in mortality of 24% (AHA & ILCOR, 2000). The effect on mortality has been shown to continue for up to 10 years (Gruppo Italiano per lo Studio della Streptochinasi nell'Infarto Miocardico (GISSI),

1998). Box 11.1 lists some of the thrombolytic drugs that are available.

The onset of pain to the commencement of thrombolytic therapy is a major determinant of myocardial salvage and long term prognosis (GISSI, 1998).

'Time is muscle'. The earlier therapy is started, the more effective it will be. Box 11.2 lists the recommended indications for thrombolytic therapy.

Absolute and relative contraindications for thrombolytic therapy are detailed in Box 11.3. It is important to decide whether the benefits of thrombolytic therapy outweigh the risks. In particular the size and site of infarct together with the time interval since the onset of chest pain must be taken into account.

Percutaneous transluminal coronary angioplasty (PTCA) is the recommended method for reperfusion in STEMI. It is the primary PCI if this can be achieved within 90 minutes of contact with a medical team (Resuscitation Council, (UK), 2005) as there is a

---

Box 11.1 Thrombolytic drugs

- Streptokinase
- Alteplase
- Reteplase
- Tenecteplase

(British Medical Association & Royal Pharmaceutical Society of Great Britain, 2008)

Box 11.2 Indications for thrombolytic therapy

- Acute myocardial infarction when benefit outweighs the risk of treatment
- Greatest benefit in patients with ST segment elevation (particularly anterior myocardial infarction and in patients with bundle branch block)
- <12 hours of the onset of symptoms (ideally within 1 hour) (alteplase, reteplase and streptokinase); >12 hours of the onset of symptoms, specialist advice should be sought. Tenecteplase is usually administered within 6 hours of the onset of symptoms

(British Medical Association & Royal Pharmaceutical Society of Great Britain, 2008)

> **Box 11.3** Contraindications for thrombolytic therapy
>
> - Recent haemorrhage, trauma or surgery
> - Coagulation defects
> - Bleeding diatheses
> - Oesophageal varices
> - History of cerebrovascular disease (especially recent events or residual disability)
> - Coma
> - Aortic dissection
> - Aneurysm
> - Recent symptoms of peptic ulceration
> - Severe hypertension
> - Previous anaphylaxis to streptokinase
> - Heavy vaginal bleeding
> - Active pulmonary disease with cavitation
> - Acute pancreatitis, pericarditis, bacterial endocarditis and severe hepatic disease
>
> N.B. Streptokinase cannot be repeated >4 days following first administration.
> (British Medical Association & Royal Pharmaceutical Society of Great Britain, 2008)

lower risk of bleeding than with thrombolytic therapy. Coronary angiography is performed via the femoral artery to identify the culprit lesion within in the occluded coronary artery. Then a guide wire is passed distally to the thrombus allowing a deflated balloon to be positioned at the site of the lesion; it is then is inflated to reopen the artery. Often a stent is positioned simultaneously to reduce restenosis at the point where the thrombus occurred.

Although an effective method of coronary reperfusion, PTCA is not universally available. It requires a staffed catheter laboratory, together with an operator skilled in the technique of PCI, available 24 hours a day (Resuscitation Council (UK), 2006). If there is any likelihood of a delay in a patient undergoing primary PCI then thrombolytic therapy must be considered as a method of ensuring coronary reperfusion.

Chapter summary

Patients presenting with ACS require urgent assessment and investigations to help confirm the diagnosis and establish the immediate risk. The appropriate immediate treatment should be promptly started and its effect evaluated.

References

Ambrose J, Fuster V (1997) Can we predict future acute coronary events in patients with stable coronary artery disease? (editorial; comment). *Journal of the American Medical Association* **277**:343–4.

American Heart Association (AHA) & International Liaison Committee on Resuscitation (2000) Guidelines 2000 for Cardiopulmonary Resuscitation and Emergency Cardiovascular Care – an international consensus on science. *Resuscitation* **46**:1–448.

British Medical Association & Royal Pharmaceutical Society of Great Britain (2008) *BNF 55*. BMJ, London.

Burke A, Farb A, Malcom G *et al.* (1999) Plaque rupture and sudden death related to exertion in men with coronary artery disease. *Journal of the American Medical Association* **281**:921–6.

Chesebro J, Rauch U, Fuster V, Badimon J (1997) Pathogenesis of thrombosis in coronary artery disease. *Haemostasis* **27**(suppl 1):12–18.

Gruppo Italiano per lo Studio della Streptochinasi nell'Infarto Miocardico (GISSI) (1998) Ten year follow-up of the first megatrial testing thrombolytic therapy in patients with acute myocardial infarction: results of the GISSI study. *Circulation* **98**:2659–65.

ISIS 1 (1986) Randomised trial of intravenous atenolol among 16,027 cases of suspected myocardial infarction ISIS 1. *Lancet* **2**:57–66.

ISIS 2 (1988) Randomised trial of intravenous streptokinase, oral aspirin, both, or neither among 17,187 cases of suspected acute myocardial infarction: ISIS-2. ISIS-2 (Second International Study of Infarct Survival) Collaborative Group. *Lancet* **13**(2):349–60.

Kong D, Califf R, Miller D *et al.* (1998) Clinical outcomes of therapeutic agents that block the platelet glycoprotein 11b/111a integrin in ischaemic heart disease. *Circulation* **98**:2829–35.

Maroko P, Radvany P, Braunwald E, Hale S (1975) Reduction of infarct size by oxygen inhalation following acute coronary occlusion. *Circulation* **52**:360–8.

Resuscitation Council (UK) (2006) *Advanced Life Support*, 5th Ed. Resuscitation Council (UK), London.

Chapter 12

Management of Peri-Arrest Arrhythmias

Introduction

The term peri-arrest arrhythmias is used to describe cardiac arrhythmias that precede cardiac arrest or complicate the early post-resuscitation period (Colquhoun & Vincent, 2004). If untreated, they may lead to cardiac arrest or potentially avoidable deterioration in the patient (Resuscitation Council (UK), 2006). Ventricular fibrillation is often triggered by a tachyarrhythmia.

A successful strategy to reduce the mortality and morbidity of cardiac arrest must therefore include the effective management of peri-arrest arrhythmias. The Resuscitation Council (UK) provides guidance for the effective and safe management of bradycardias and tachyacardias (Resuscitation Council (UK), 2006).

The aim of this chapter is to understand the principles of the management of peri-arrest arrhythmias.

Learning outcomes

At the end of the chapter the reader will be able to:

- Discuss the principles of the use of the peri-arrest algorithms
- List the adverse clinical signs that may be associated with peri-arrest arrhythmias
- Discuss the treatment options
- Outline the management of bradycardia
- Outline the management of tachycardia

Principles of the use of the peri-arrest algorithms

The Resuscitation Council (UK)'s algorithms for the management of peri-arrest arrhythmias are designed for the non-specialist advanced life support (ALS) provider in order to provide effective and safe treatment in the emergency situation (Resuscitation Council (UK), 2006). The following points regarding the use of the algorithms need emphasising:

- They are specifically designed for the peri-arrest situation and are not intended to encompass all clinical situations
- The arrows indicate progression from one stage of treatment to the next, only if the cardiac arrhythmia persists
- Important variables, which can influence the management, include the arrhythmia itself, the haemodynamic status of the patient, local procedures and local circumstances/facilities
- Stated drug doses are based on average body weight and may therefore need adjustment in some situations
- Anti-arrhythmic strategies can cause cardiac arrhythmias; clinical deterioration may result from the treatment itself rather than a consequence of its lack of effect
- High dose of a single anti-arrhythmic drug or use of different drugs can cause hypotension and myocardial depression
- Expert help must be summoned early if simple measures are ineffective

(Colquhoun & Vincent, 2004)

Adverse clinical signs associated with peri-arrest arrhythmias

The treatment for most peri-arrest arrhythmias will be dependent upon the presence or absence of certain adverse clinical signs:

- *Clinical evidence of low cardiac output*: e.g. hypotension, impaired consciousness (reduced cerebral perfusion), pallor, cold and clammy extremities
- *Excessive tachycardia*: (typically >150/minute) leads to a shortened diastole, which can result in a fall in cardiac output and reduced coronary blood flow (causing myocardial ischaemia)

- *Excessive bradycardia*: usually <40/minute, though higher rates may not be tolerated by some patients
- *Heart failure*: pulmonary oedema (left ventricular failure) or raised jugular venous pressure and hepatic engorgement (right ventricular failure)
- *Chest pain*: more likely to be associated with a tachyarrhythmia than a bradyarrhythmia; suggests myocardial ischaemia

(Resuscitation Council (UK), 2006)

Management of bradycardia

Bradycardia is defined as a ventricular rate <60/minute. An absolute rate below this level can be easily recognised. However it is also important to identify patients with clinical evidence of critically low cardiac output in whom rates >60/minute are inappropriately slow; this is termed relative bradycardia (Colquhoun & Vincent, 2004). The Resuscitation Council (UK) bradycardia algorithm is detailed in Figure 12.1.

- Assess the patient following the ABCDE approach (Chapter 3)
- Administer high-concentration oxygen
- Commence ECG monitoring and secure intravenous access; ideally record a 12-lead electrocardiogram (ECG)
- Ascertain whether there are any adverse clinical signs (Box 12.1)
- If adverse clinical signs are present (i.e. immediate treatment required), administer atropine 500 µg IV; this may be repeated up to a maximum of 3 mg (Resuscitation Council (UK), 2006)
- If adverse clinical signs are not present or if the administration of atropine is effective, subsequent treatment should then be

---

Box 12.1 Bradycardia: adverse clinical signs

Systolic blood pressure <90 mmHg
Ventricular rate <40/minute
Ventricular arrhythmias compromising the blood pressure
Heart failure
Altered conscious level, e.g. drowsiness

If appropriate, give oxygen, cannulate a vein and record a 12-lead ECG

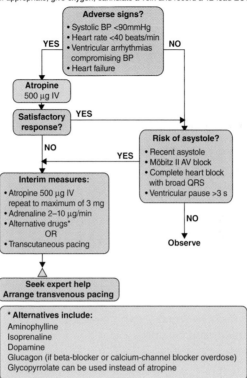

Fig. 12.1 Bradycardia algorithm. Includes rates inappropriately slow for haemodynamic state. Reproduced with permission of Resuscitation Council (UK).

guided by the presence or absence of risk factors for asystole (Box 12.2) (Colquhoun & Vincent, 2004)

If there has not been a satisfactory response to atropine 500 µg IV or if there is a risk factor for asystole (Box 12.2), the definitive treatment is transvenous pacing. While waiting for expert help, possible interim measures include:

- Atropine 500 µg IV repeated at a few minute intervals to a maximum of 3 mg (Colquhoun & Vincent, 2004)
- Transcutaneous or external pacing (Falk *et al.*, 1983)

Box 12.2 Bradycardia: risk factors for asystole

Recent asystole
Second-degree AV block Mobitz type II
Third-degree (complete) AV block, particularly if broad QRS complex or if
heart rate <40/minute
Ventricular standstill (pause) >3 seconds

Box 12.3 Tachycardia: adverse clinical signs

Systolic blood pressure <90 mmHg
Heart rate >150/minute
Heart failure
Altered conscious level, e.g. drowsiness
Chest pain

- Adrenaline infusion 2–10 µg/minute titrated to response (1 ml of 1:1000 adrenaline in 500 ml of 0.9% normal saline; rate 1–5 ml/minute) – usually only used if transcutaneous pacing is not immediately available
- Fist pacing

Management of a tachycardia

The Resuscitation Council (UK) tachycardia algorithm is detailed in Figure 12.2.

- Assess the patient following the ABCDE approach (Chapter 3)
- Administer high-concentration oxygen
- Commence ECG monitoring and secure intravenous access; ideally record a 12-lead ECG
- Ascertain whether there are any adverse clinical signs (Box 12.3)
- If adverse clinical signs are present (i.e. immediate treatment required), perform synchronised electrical cardioversion. If this is unsuccessful, administer amiodarone 300 mg IV over 10–20 minutes, followed by 900 mg over 24 hours (Resuscitation Council (UK), 2006)

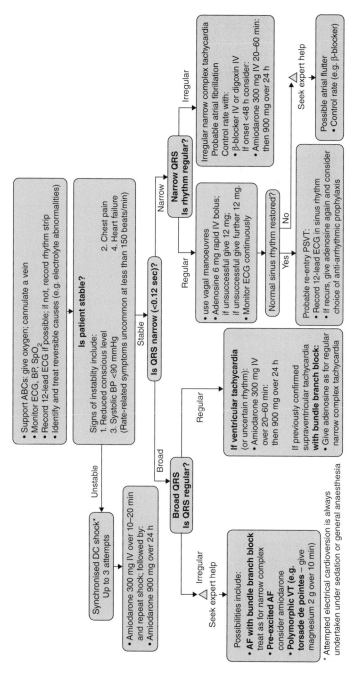

Fig. 12.2 Tachycardia algorithm (with pulse). Reproduced with permission of Resuscitation Council (UK).

- If adverse clinical signs are not present, ascertain whether the QRS complex is narrow (<3 small squares or 0.12 secs) or broad, regular or irregular

Regular narrow complex tachycardia

> It is important to exclude sinus tachycardia which is likely to be regular, with a rate <140/minute and non-paroxysmal, i.e. it does not start and end abruptly. The treatment for sinus tachycardia is targeted at identifying and treating the cause (where appropriate).

- If there are no contra-indications, try vagal manoeuvres (Box 12.4). They are used to stimulate the vagus nerve and induce a reflex slowing of the heart (Smith, 2003). They are successful in terminating 25% of narrow complex tachycardias (Resuscitation Council (UK), 2006). Caution should be exercised regarding the use of vagal manoeuvres. Profound vagal tone can induce sudden bradycardia and trigger ventricular fibrillation, particularly in the presence of digitalis toxicity or acute cardiac ischaemia (Colquhoun & Vincent, 2004)
- If vagal manoeuvres fail, and the arrhythmia is not atrial flutter, administer adenosine 6 mg IV (rapid bolus); if there is no response administer adenosine 12 mg IV (rapid bolus) and again if there is no response administer a further 12 mg dose (Resuscitation Council (UK), 2006).
- If both vagal manoeuvres and adenosine are unsuccessful, seek expert help
- If the arrhythmia is atrial flutter, seek expert help

Box 12.4 Vagal manoeuvres

Carotid sinus massage – should not be used in the presence of a carotid bruit as atheromatous plaque rupture could embolise into the cerebral circulation causing a cerebral vascular accident; elderly patients are more vulnerable to plaque rupture and cerebral vascular complications (Bastuli & Orlowski, 1985; Skinner & Vincent, 1997)

Valsalva manoeuvre – forced expiration against a closed glottis, e.g. ask the patient to blow into a 20 ml syringe with enough force to push the plunger back (Resuscitation Council (UK), 2006)

Irregular narrow complex tachycardia

An irregular narrow complex tachycardia is likely to be atrial fibrillation or, rarely, atrial flutter with varying atrioventricular (AV) block; record a 12-lead ECG to assist in interpretation (Resuscitation Council (UK), 2006).

If there are no adverse signs present, treatment options are:

- Drug therapy to control the ventricular rate, e.g. beta-blocker, digoxin or diltazem
- Drug therapy to control the rhythm (chemical cardioversion)
- Synchronised electrical cardioversion to control the rhythm
- Treatment to prevent complications such as anti-coagulation

(Nolan *et al.*, 2005)

Seek expert help to establish the most appropriate treatment for the patient. The longer the patient remains in atrial fibrillation, the greater the risk of an atrial blood clot developing; therefore:

- *Duration of atrial fibrillation >48 hours*: if rhythm control (chemical or electrical cardioversion) is indicated, it is usual practice for patients to be fully coagulated first or the presence of an atrial clot to be excluded by transoesphageal echocardiography before treatment
- *Duration of atrial fibrillation <48 hours*: if rhythm control is indicated, amiodarone 300 mg IV over 20–60 minutes, followed by 900 mg IV over 24 hours is recommended (synchronised electrical cardioversion remains a treatment option in these patients: it is more successful than chemical cardioversion at restoring sinus rhythm)

(Nolan *et al.*, 2005)

Regular broad complex tachycardia

A regular broad complex tachycardia is regular is likely to be ventricular tachycardia (i.e. ventricular in origin) (Colquhoun & Vincent, 2004); if there are no adverse signs, administer amiodarone 300 mg IV over 20–60 minutes, followed by an infusion of 900 mg over 24 hours (Resuscitation Council (UK), 2006).

If there is a regular broad complex tachycardia that is considered to be supraventricular tachycardia with bundle branch block (rare), follow the protocol for regular narrow complex tachycardia described above, i.e. adenosine etc.

Irregular broad complex tachycardia

Seek expert help.
An irregular broad complex tachycardia could be:

- *Atrial fibrillation with bundle branch block* (most common cause): treat as for atrial fibrillation (irregular narrow complex tachycardia) (see above)
- *Atrial fibrillation in the presence of Wolf Parkinson Syndrome* (pre-excitation) – greater variation in the morphology (shape) and width of the QRS complexes compared to atrial fibrillation with bundle branch block: avoid adenosine, digoxin, verapamil and diltiazem as these drugs block the AV junction which can cause an increase in pre-excitation; synchronised electrical cardioversion is usually the safest treatment option
- *Polymorphic ventricular tachycardia* e.g. torsades de points: stop all medications that can cause a prolonged QT interval, correct any electrolyte abnormalities and administer magnesium sulphate 2 mg (8 mmol) IV over 10 minutes; overdrive cardiac pacing is sometimes required

(Nolan *et al.*, 2005)

Chapter summary

A successful strategy to reduce the mortality and morbidity of cardiac arrest must include the effective management of peri-arrest arrhythmias. In this chapter the Resuscitation Council (UK) guidelines for the management of bradycardias and tachycardias have been outlined. Always seek expert help when necessary.

References

Bastuli J, Orlowski J (1985) Stroke as a complication of carotid sinus massage. *Critical Care Medicine* **13**:869.

Colquhoun M, Vincent R (2004) Management of peri-arrest arrhythmias. In: Colquhoun M *et al.* (eds) *ABC of Resuscitation*, 5th Ed. BMJ Books, London.

Falk R, Zoll P, Zoll R (1983) Safety and efficacy of noninvasive pacing. *New England Journal of Medicine* **309**:1166–8.

Nolan J, Deakin C, Soar J *et al.* (2005) European Resuscitation Council Guidelines for Resuscitation 2005: Section 4. Adult advanced life support. *Resuscitation* **675S**:S39–S86.

Resuscitation Council (UK) (2006) *Advanced Life Support*, 5th Ed. Resuscitation Council (UK), London.

Skinner D, Vincent R (1997) *Cardiopulmonary Resuscitation*, 2nd Ed. Oxford University Press, Oxford.

Smith G (2003) *ALERT Acute Life-Threatening Events Recognition and Treatment*, 2nd Ed. University of Portsmouth, Portsmouth.

Chapter 13

Post-Resuscitation Care

Jagtar Singh Pooni

Introduction

The goal of resuscitation is to produce a patient with normal cerebral function, a stable cardiac output, a stable electrocardiogram (ECG) and adequate organ perfusion (European Resuscitation Council, 1998). However complete recovery from a cardiopulmonary arrest is rarely immediate and the return of a spontaneous circulation (ROSC) is just the start, and not the end, of a successful cardiopulmonary resuscitation (CPR).

Following ROSC, patients may exhibit a wide spectrum of physiological states; some will fully recover with normal haemodynamic and cerebral function, while others will remain comatose with cardiorespiratory dysfunction. All patients will require careful and ongoing assessment to determine the status of vital functions. The ABCDE approach to the assessment of the critically ill patient (see Chapter 3) is recommended. Once the patient has been stabilised, transfer to definitive care will need to be arranged.

The aim of this chapter is to understand the principles of post-resuscitation care.

Learning objectives

At the end of the chapter the reader will be able to:

- List the goals of post-resuscitation care
- Outline the initial assessment priorities (ABCDE approach)
- Discuss transfer to definitive care
- Describe measures to limit damage to vital organs
- Predict non-survivors

Goals of post-resuscitation care

The goals of post resuscitation care are to:

- Perform an initial assessment of the patient's vital signs and prevent a further cardiac arrest
- Transfer the patient to definitive care (usually intensive care unit (ICU) or coronary care unit (CCU))
- Limit damage to vital organs
- Predict non-survivors

(European Resuscitation Council, 1998)

Initial assessment priorities

The ABCDE approach to patient assessment and treatment (see Chapter 3) is recommended in the immediate post-resuscitation period (Resuscitation Council (UK), 2006).

Airway

The patient's airway is usually impaired following a cardiac arrest. Look, listen and feel for the signs of airway obstruction (see Chapter 6), in particular listen for:

- *Gurgling*: indicates the presence of fluid, e.g. secretions or vomit, in the mouth or upper airway; apply suction using a wide-bore rigid Yankeur catheter, use a flexible catheter if suctioning down an oropharyngeal airway or tracheal tube
- *Snoring*: indicates that the pharynx is being partially obstructed by the tongue; position the patient in a lateral position, insert an airway device if necessary (see Chapter 6)

If the patient is unable to maintain his own airway, the anaesthetist may decide to insert a tracheal tube.

Breathing

Prolonged hypoxia and inadequate ventilation will increase the risk of a further cardiac arrest and could contribute to further cerebral injury (Resuscitation Council (UK), 2006). It is important to check whether the patient is breathing adequately or not. Look, listen and feel to assess breathing:

Count the respiratory rate

Evaluate chest movement: in particular check for symmetrical chest movement; if ribs have been fractured during chest compressions, there may be a pneumothorax or a flail segment (Resuscitation Council (UK), 2006). Request a chest radiograph.

Commence pulse oximetry and note the oxygen saturation reading (Figure 13.1).

Undertake arterial blood gas anlysis (Figure 13.2).

Check the position of the trachea: place the tip of the index finger into the supersternal notch, let it slip either side of the trachea and determine whether it fits more easily into one or other side of the trachea (Ford *et al.*, 2005). Deviation of the trachea to one side indicates mediastinal shift (e.g. pneumothorax, lung fibrosis or pleural fluid).

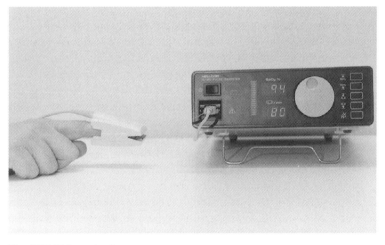

Fig. 13.1 Pulse oximetry.

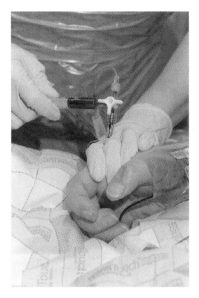

Fig. 13.2 Arterial blood sampling.

Palpate the chest wall: to detect surgical emphysema or crepitus (suggesting a pneumothorax *until* proven otherwise) (Smith, 2003).

Perform chest percussion:

• Place the left hand on the patient's chest wall. Ensure the fingers are slightly separated, with the middle finger pressed firmly into the intercostal space to be percussed (Ford *et al.*, 2005)

• Strike the centre of the middle phalanx of the middle finger sharply using the tip of the middle finger of the right hand (Ford *et al.*, 2005) (Figure 13.3). Deliver the stroke using a quick flick of the wrist and finger joints not from the arm or shoulder. The percussing finger should be bent so that its terminal phalanx is at right angles to the metacarpal bones when the blow is delivered, and it strikes the percussed finger in a perpendicular way. The percussing finger should then be removed immediately, like a clapper inside a bell, otherwise the resultant sound will be dampened (Epstein *et al.*, 2003)

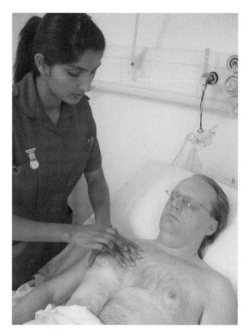

Fig. 13.3 Chest percussion.

- Percuss the anterior and lateral chest wall. Percuss the from side to side, and top to bottom, comparing both sides and looking for asymmetry
- Categorise the percussion sounds (see below)
- If an area of altered resonance is located, map out its boundaries by percussing from areas of normal to altered resonance (Ford *et al.*, 2005)
- Sit the patient forward and then percuss the posterior chest wall, omitting the areas covered by the scapulae. Ask the patient to move his elbows forward across the front of his chest: this will rotate the scapulae anteriorly and out of the way (Talley & O'Connor, 2001). It may be helpful to offer the patient a pillow to lean on
- Again percuss from side to side, and top to bottom, comparing both sides and looking for asymmetry. Don't forget that the lungs extend much further down posteriorly than anteriorly (Epstein *et al.*, 2003)
- Categorise the percussion sounds (see below)

(Source: Jevon, 2006)

Causes of different percussion notes:

- *Resonant*: air-filled lung
- *Dull*: liver, spleen, heart, lug consolidation/collapse
- *Stony dull*: pleural effusion/thickening
- *Hyper-resonant*: pneumothorax, emphysema
- *Tympanitic*: gas-filled viscus

(Ford *et al.*, 2005)

Auscultate the chest:

- If appropriate, ask the patient to breathe in and out normally through his mouth
- Auscultate the anterior chest from side to side, and top to bottom. Auscultate over equivalent areas and compare the volume and character of the sounds and note any additional sounds. Compare the sounds during inspiration and expiration
- Auscultate the posterior chest, from side to side, and top to bottom (Figure 13.4). Auscultate over equivalent areas and compare the volume and character of the sounds and note any additional sounds. Compare the sounds during inspiration and expiration
- Note the location and quality of the sounds heard

(Jevon & Cunnington, 2006)

Evaluate air entry, the depth of breathing and the equality of breath sounds on both sides of the chest. Bronchial breathing indicates lung consolidation; absent or reduced sounds suggest a pneumothorax or pleural fluid (Smith, 2003). In particular, note any additional breath sounds:

- *Wheezes (rhonchi)*: high-pitched musical sounds associated with air being forced through narrowed airways, e.g. asthma (Ford *et al.*, 2005). They are usually more pronounced on expiration. Inspiratory wheeze (stridor) is usually indicative of severe upper airway obstruction, e.g. foreign body, laryngeal oedema. If both inspiratory and expiratory wheezes are heard, this is usually due to excessive airway secretions (Adam & Osborne, 2005)

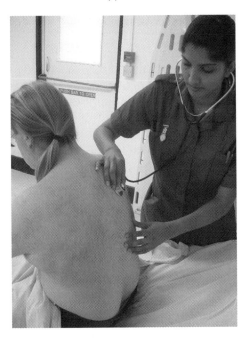

Fig. 13.4 Chest auscultation.

- *Crackles (crepitations)*: non-musical sounds associated with reopening of a collapsed airway, e.g. pulmonary oedema (Ford *et al.*, 2005). Crackles are usually localised in pneumonia and mild cases of bronchiectasis; in pulmonary oedema and fibrosing alveolitis, both lung bases are equally affected (Epstein *et al.*, 2003)
- *Pleural friction rub*: leathery/creaking sounds during inspiration and expiration, evident in areas of inflammation when the normally smooth pleural surfaces are roughened and rub on each other (Adam & Osborne, 2005)

If not already done, a tracheal tube may need to be inserted. This will secure the airway and facilitate mechanical ventilation if required. Correct tracheal tube placement should be verified. Coughing on the tracheal tube will result in increased catecholamine levels which could induce cardiac arrhythmias and/ or hypertension (Resuscitation Council (UK), 2006). If this occurs, a decision will need to be made, usually by the anaesthetist, on whether to remove the tracheal tube or sedate the patient and leave it *in situ*.

If the patient is not breathing, mechanical ventilation should continue using available equipment, e.g. bag/valve device, portable ventilator. If the patient is breathing adequately, high concentrations of oxygen should be administered via a non-rebreathe mask. Continue oxygen saturation monitoring and perform regular arterial blood gas analysis.

A nasogastric tube may need to be inserted to decompress the stomach (gastric inflation is often associated with bag/valve/mask ventilation and can cause diaphragmatic splinting) and allow aspiration of gastric contents.

Circulation

Following ROSC, the cardiac rhythm and haemodynamic function are likely to be unstable. Cardiac arrhythmias are common, varied and often transient. Continuous ECG monitoring is essential and anti-arrhythmic therapy may be required. Electrolyte levels should be checked and any abnormalities treated. A 12-lead ECG should be recorded. If a patient with a classical history of myocardial infarction has ECG changes suggestive of acute ischaemia, immediate referral for either thrombolytic therapy or emergency percutaneous coronary intervention should be made.

Accurate haemodynamic monitoring will be required. The pulse and blood pressure should be monitored, together with adequacy of peripheral perfusion (temperature, colour and capillary refill). The insertion of an arterial cannula will allow continuous arterial blood pressure measurements and repeated sampling for arterial blood gas analysis.

Central venous pressure monitoring may be required and urine output should be closely monitored. A pulmonary artery catheter probe may sometimes be inserted, though non-invasive Doppler techniques may be a better alternative. Fluids and inotropes may be required depending on haemodynamic measurements.

Neurological assessment

A baseline neurological assessment should be undertaken and documented using the Glasgow Coma Score (Figure 13.5). This

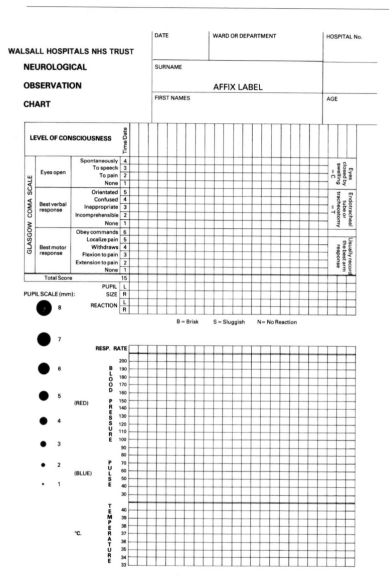

Fig. 13.5 Glasgow Coma Scale incorporated in a neurological observation chart (Reproduced with permission of Walsall Hospitals NHS Trust).

score will provide a bench mark for further recordings. In the post-resuscitation phase, pupil size is a poor prognostic indicator because it can be affected by carbon dioxide retention, atropine, adrenaline and local ischaemia to the front of the eye.

Investigations

It is important to ascertain the cause of the cardiopulmonary arrest. The patient's history and events leading up to the cardiopulmonary arrest may be significant. A number of investigations will need to be carried out, these are summarised in Figure 13.6.

Transfer to definitive care

It is important to facilitate the safe transfer of the patient between the site of resuscitation and an appropriate place for definitive care (Resuscitation Council (UK), 2006). This will usually either be CCU or ICU (Figure 13.7). If the patient is breathing spontaneously and does not require multi-organ support, transfer to CCU is usually arranged. Indications for transfer to the ICU include:

- Requirement for continued intubation either for protection of the airway or mechanical ventilation
- Haemodynamic instability requiring invasive monitoring and pharmacological or mechanical support
- Requirement for multi-organ support

Transfer can be hazardous; a portable monitor/defibrillator together with airway, ventilation and suction equipment, the necessary drugs and senior personnel should accompany the patient (Skinner & Vincent, 1997).

Full blood count
Biochemistry (urea and electrolytes, glucose, cardiac enzymes)
12-lead ECG
Chest radiography
Arterial blood gas analysis

Fig. 13.6 Post-resuscitation care investigations.

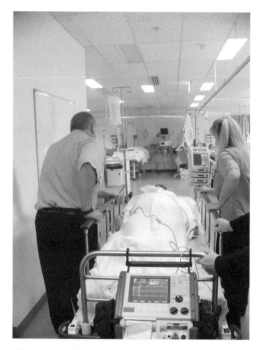

Fig. 13.7 Transfer to intensive care unit.

In their publication *Transport of the Critically Ill Adult Patient*, The Intensive Care Society (2002) has made recommendations for the organisation and clinical provision of transfers.

Measures to limit damage to vital organs

Myocardial function

As an adequate coronary perfusion pressure is essential to oxygenate the myocardium, it is important to ascertain the patient's 'normal blood pressure' and avoid hypotension (European Resuscitation Council, 1998).

If the cardiac arrest was precipitated by an acute myocardial infarction, thrombolytic therapy to restore coronary artery patency should be considered (Gershlick & More, 1998). However it is generally accepted that thrombolysis should not be administered if CPR has been vigorous (Skinner & Vincent, 1997). If available, angioplasty may be beneficial.

Neurological function

Vigilant attention to the details of oxygenation and cerebral perfusion following resuscitation can significantly minimise the risk of secondary neurological injury and maximise the likelihood of full neurological recovery (American Heart Association (AHA) & International Liaison Committee on Resuscitation (ILCOR), 2000).

As normal cerebral autoregulation is lost following a period of global ischaemia, cerebral perfusion pressure is reliant upon mean arterial pressure (Kagstrom *et al.*, 1983). If mean arterial blood pressure falls, or if intracranial pressure rises, cerebral perfusion pressure may decrease which could further compromise cerebral blood flow (AHA & ILCOR, 2000) and worsen neurological injury.

The patient's mean arterial blood pressure should therefore be closely monitored, with inotropes and fluids administered if necessary (European Resuscitation Council, 1998). In addition, care should be taken to avoid a rise in intracranial pressure, e.g. during tracheal suction. The head should be maintained in a mid-line position and elevated to approximately 30 degrees to facilitate venous drainage (AHA & ILCOR, 2000).

There is no evidence that barbiturates and calcium channel blockers are neuroprotective (Brain Resuscitation Clinical Trial 1 Study Group, 1986; Brain Resuscitation Clinical Trial 11 Study Group, 1991).

There is evidence that sustained hypocapnoea (low PCO_2) could worsen cerebral ischaemia (Ausina *et al.*, 1998). Hyperventilation in the post-resuscitation period should therefore be avoided.

Convulsions, which occur in approximately 5–15% of post-cardiac arrest patients (Roine *et al.*, 1990), can increase cerebral metabolism by 300–400% (Siesjo, 1978). As convulsions could impair cerebral recovery, they should be controlled with, for example, benzodiazepines, barbiturates or phenytoin (European Resuscitation Council, 1998).

Renal function

Urine output is a good indicator of renal perfusion. Patients who have had prolonged CPR and a long period of hypotension commonly develop acute tubular necrosis (European Resuscitation Council, 1998). Protection of renal function is best achieved by adequate intravenous fluid filling and maintenance of an adequate perfusion pressure, i.e. usually a mean arterial pressure in excess of 70 mmHg. Central venous pressure monitoring is usually required. Following CPR, most patients will therefore need to be catheterised and hourly urine output measurements undertaken.

Low-dose dopamine does not provide specific renal protection and is therefore no longer indicated in acute oliguric renal failure (Marik & Iglesias, 1999). Also, the use of diuretics does not provide protection of renal function.

Metabolic function

Blood glucose levels should be closely monitored as cerebral injury can cause them to rise; hyperglycaemia should be avoided as it will increase cerebral metabolism. This may have detrimental effects on neurological outcome (Pulsineli *et al.*, 1982). Hypoglycaemia should also be avoided as it can have detrimental effects on cerebral blood flow autoregulation and membrane stability (Ceber *et al.*, 1990).

Metabolic acidosis usually develops during a cardiac arrest resulting in low pH (acidaemia), low bicarbonate and a base deficit; the normal physiological response is an increase in minute ventilation (respiratory compensation) (Resuscitation Council (UK), 2006). Blood gas and acid–base abnormalities should be controlled by adequate ventilation and restoration of renal function.

The routine use of sodium bicarbonate to treat acidosis is no longer recommended, except in certain situations, e.g. tricyclic overdose, hyperkalaemia and profound acidaemia (pH <7.1, base deficit >10) (Resuscitation Council (UK), 2006). If it is used, adequate ventilation is essential to avoid respiratory acidosis (the bicarbonate ion is excreted as carbon dioxide via the lungs). The blood pH and base excess should also be measured.

Temperature control and therapeutic hypothermia

Pyrexia will cause an increase in the cerebral metabolic rate (8% for every 1 °C rise in temperature) which could create an imbalance between oxygen demand and oxygen supply (European Resuscitation Council, 1998). Following resuscitation, even a modest increase in temperature could increase the cerebral metabolic rate sufficiently to impair cerebral recovery (Minamisawa *et al.*, 1990). In the post-resuscitation period pyrexia should therefore be aggressively treated (AHA & ILCOR, 2000).

Induced hypothermia is used effectively during certain surgical procedures, e.g. cardiac surgery. Evidence has emerged that hypothermia is beneficial in the post-resuscitation period, especially for patients who have had an out of hospital cardiac arrest (Bernard *et al.*, 2002; Holzer, 2002). These two randomised controlled studies have shown that induced hypothermia leads to improved neurological outcome compared with groups treated without hypothermia. Hypothermia limits the anoxic neurological injury and this translates into improved survival.

Indeed, after resuscitation to a stable cardiac rhythm and cardiac output, the brain is the organ that influences the individual's survival most significantly. The cause of death of over 60% of those patients dying following successful resuscitation after an out of hospital cardiac arrest is neurological injury. Approximately 25% of those dying after resuscitation following a cardiac arrest in hospital also die from neurological injury. This underlines the importance of preventing or limiting neurological injury in post-resuscitation care.

Indeed, ILCOR (2003) recommends that 'unconscious adult patients with spontaneous circulation after out of hospital cardiac arrest should be cooled to 32 °C–34 °C for 12–24 hours when the initial rhythm was ventricular fibrillation and that such cooling may also be beneficial for other rhythms or in-hospital cardiac arrests'.

Previously, post-resuscitation care was supportive but now, with therapeutic hypothermia, active management should be used to limit neurological injury and so improve survival. The mechanism of action is not fully understood. Neuro-protection may be achieved by:

- Reduction in cerebral metabolism
- Prevention of cerebral vasodialation. The reduction in intracranial pressure could improve cerebral blood flow
- Suppression of the inflammatory cascade
- Decreased radical formation
- Improved ionic homeostasis

The techniques used for induced hypothermia include:

- Antipyretics, e.g. paracetamol
- Fans
- Ice packs to axillae, groin and major vessels
- Cold fluids. Crystalloid solutions at 30 ml/kg at 4 °C infused over 30 minutes
- Water-filled blankets – temperature regulated
- Forced cold air
- Cardiopulmonary bypass
- Purpose-made cooling devices (Figure 13.8)

Hypothermia should be started as soon as possible, aiming for a temperature of 32–34 °C, and continued for 12–24 hours. Local guidelines (Figure 13.9) will determine which patients should have induced hypothermia following cardiac resuscitation, and

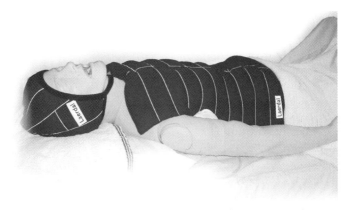

Fig. 13.8 Cooling device. Reproduced with permission from Laerdal Medical Ltd, Orpington, Kent, (UK).

Introduction and background

Patients admitted to hospital following resuscitation from an out of hospital cardiac arrest have high mortality and risk of neurological injury. Induction of mild hypothermia (32–34 °C) in adult patients, who have sustained out of hospital ventricular fibrillation (VF)/pulseless ventricular tachycardia (VT) and recovered spontaneous circulation but not consciousness, has been shown to significantly improve mortality and neurological outcome.

Recent randomized controlled trials (Bernard *et al.*, 2002; Holzer, 2002), systematic reviews and meta-analysis (Holzer & Bernard, 2005; Cheumg *et al.*, 2006) have confirmed the efficacy of therapeutic hypothermia.

Inclusion criteria

- Witnessed cardiac arrest (VF/VT) with ROSC
- Persistent Glasgow coma score <8
- Blood pressure maintained with or without vasopressors after CPR
- No other cause of coma

Exclusion criteria

- Absolute:
  ○ Do not actively rescuscitate (DNAR) order in place
  ○ Cardiogenic shock
  ○ Multiple organ failure
  ○ Children under 16
  ○ Pregnancy

- Relative:
  ○ Major head trauma
  ○ Recent major surgery within 14 days
  ○ Systemic infection/sepsis
  ○ Other causes of coma (drug intoxication, pre-existing coma prior to cardiac arrest)
  ○ Known bleeding diathesis

Fig. 13.9 Therapeutic hypothermia guidelines (Reproduced with kind permission from Dr Shameer Gopal, Consultant in Anaesthesia and Intensive Care Medicine, The Royal Wolverhampton Hospitals NHS Trust).

Eligibility for admission to the critical care unit for cooling must be confirmed by the consultant intensivist on-call.

Aims

- Cool to a target temperature of 32–34 °C for 24 hours
- Target time to reach the temperature: 6–8 hours
- Rewarm after a period of 24 hours to normothermia

(The 24 hour time period is from the time of initiation of cooling)

Time cooling commenced:	Time desired temperature achieved:	Time rewarming started:

Cooling

Methods

External cooling with cooling blankets and ice (eligibility confirmed and materials gathered; record baseline core temperature):

- Sandwich the patient with two cooling blankets
- Sedation using propofol and alfentanil
- Paralysis using atracurium/cisatracurium infusion
- Place an arterial line
- Ice packs in groin, chest, axilla and side of neck
- Cold saline infusion via peripheral line/femoral line (30 ml/ kg of 4 °C normal saline over 30 minutes)
- Monitor vitals signs and arrhythmias

External cooling with Arctic Sun Vest device:

- Effective for patients with body surface area less than 2.4 m²
- Cool patients using pads after connecting to the device
- Set target temperature. Sedate and paralyse as above
- These pads can be used with external pacing pads

Fig. 13.9 *Continued*

Maintenenance of hypothermia and supportive therapy

- Continuous temperature monitoring (bladder probe, nasopharyngeal probe)
- Aim for a mean arterial pressure of 70 mmHg (dependent on urine output)
- Sedate, paralyse and ventilate
- Regular arterial blood gas measurements. Maintain carbon dioxide between 4 and 4.5 kPa, $PaO_2 > 13$ kPa
- Monitor electrolytes (magnesium and potassium), blood glucose, full blood count and coagulation profile at 12 and 24 hours
- Chest radiograph on commencement and after rewarming
- Blood cultures at 12 hours after the initiation of cooling
- Skin care every 2 hours to prevent pressure sores
- Monitor for arrhythmias, shivering, coagulopathy, hyperglycaemia, pulmonary oedema

Rewarming

Passive rewarming

This is the most critical phase as the peripheral vascular beds vasodilate and cause hypotension. Note that increase in blood lactate and metabolic acidosis may occur.

Rewarm at a rate of 0.5–1 °C/hour.

At 24 hours (after the initiation of cooling):

- Remove cooling blankets and ice
- Maintain paralysis and sedation until temperature of 36 °C is reached
- Monitor for hypotension
- Monitor for electrolyte disturbances (hyperkalemia)
- The goal after rewarming is normothermia

Controlled rewarming

The goals are the same as above.

If the Arctic Sun device is being used, the machine can be programmed for controlled rewarming over 6–8 hours. The device should be programmed to maintain a target temperature of 37 °C for the next 48 hours.

Fig. 13.9 *Continued*

by which technique. Exclusion criteria include septicaemia, multiple organ failure and cardiogenic shock. Shivering increases myocardial oxygen demand and should be promptly treated with sedation and neuromuscular blockade if required.

Core temperature should be continuously monitored by the nasopharyngeal, tympanic or bladder route. Rewarming the patient is usually by passive methods and the temperature is allowed to rise slowly. Hyperthermia, should of course be avoided.

Side effects of hypothermia include:

- Cardiovascular: decrease in cardiac output along with an increase in systemic vascular resistance. ECG changes such as J waves may occur. Below 30 °C risks of atrial fibrillation and refactory ventricular fibrillation are increased
- Respiratory: with the decrease in metabolic rate, tidal volume in mechanically ventilated patients may need to be decrease to maintain a normal $PaCO_2$
- Infection: hypothermia impairs immune function so risk of infection, e.g. pneumonia, is increased. Wound healing is impaired and there is an increased risk of pressure sores
- Metabolic: hyperglycaemia can occur due to insulin resistance. Liver enzymes and amylase may be elevated
- Renal system: diuresis may lead to electrolyte disturbances
- Acid–base: arterial blood gases are more difficult to interpret because of increased solubility of gases in hypothermia
- Haematological: impairment of coagulation and increase bleeding time can occur

Prediction of poor outcome

Predicting outcome in the immediate post-resuscitation period is fraught with difficulties; initial blood pressure measurements, pupil size and patient's age are unreliable. Approximately 80% of patients remain unconscious for varying periods of time following a successful resuscitation (Longstreth *et al.*, 1983).

Ten minutes after successful resuscitation, the lack of a pupillary response to light is a significant (>80%) indicator of poor outcome, i.e. death or vegetative state (Mullie *et al.*, 1988). Three days after a successful resuscitation, the lack of a pupillary response to light and absence of a motor response to pain are good indicators (100%) of poor outcome (Mullie *et al.*, 1988; Geocadin *et al.*, 2008).

Brain stem reflex assessment within 1 hour of successful resuscitation may help to identify patients who will not regain consciousness (Jorgensen, 1997). A Glasgow coma score of <5, 24 hours following successful resuscitation, is also a good indicator of poor outcome (Mullie *et al.*, 1988).

Chapter summary

Following ROSC, the patient must be stabilised as quickly as possible in order to try to avoid another cardiac arrest. The patient should be transferred to definitive care, usually CCU or ICU, and measures should be taken to limit damage to vital organs, including therapeutic hypothermia to limit neurological injury in accordance with local guidelines. Assessment of neurological function should be undertaken at the earliest opportunity and regularly reviewed in order to predict outcome.

References

Adam S, Osborne S (2005) *Critical Care Nursing Science and Practice*, 2nd Ed. Oxford University Press, Oxford.

American Heart Association in Collaboration with ILCOR (2000) Guidelines 2000 for Cardiopulmonary Resuscitation and Emergency Cardiovascular Care – an international consensus on science. *Resuscitation* **46**:1–448.

Ausina A, Baguena M, Nadal M *et al.* (1998) Cerebral hemodynamic changes during sustained hypocapnea in severe head injury: can hyperventilation cause cerebral ischaemia? *Acta Neurochirugica Supplement* **71**:1–4.

Bernard SA, Gray TW, Buist MD, *et al.* (2002) Treatment of comatose survivors of cardiac arrest with induced hypothermia. *New England Journal of Medicine* **346**:557–63.

Brain Resuscitation Clinical Trial 1 Study Group (1986) Randomized trial of thiopental loading in comatose survivors of cardiac arrest. *New England Journal of Medicine* **314**:397–403.

Brain Resuscitation Clinical Trial 11 Study Group (1991) A randomized clinical study of a calcium-entry blocker (lidoflazine) in the treatment of comatose survivors of cardiac arrest: *New England Journal of Medicine* **324**:1225–31.

Ceber F, Koehler R, Derrer S *et al.* (1990) Hypoglycaemia and cerebral autoregulation in anaesthetised dogs. *American Journal of Physiology* **258**:H1714–21.

Epstein O, Perkin G, Cookson J, de Bono D (2003) *Clinical examination,* 3rd Ed. Mosby London.

European Resuscitation Council (1998) *European Resuscitation Council Guidelines for Resuscitation.* Elsevier, Oxford.

Ford M, Hennessey I, Japp A (2005) *Introduction to clinical examination.* Elsevier, Oxford.

Geocadin R, Hanley D, Eleff S (2008) Post resuscitation prognostication and declaration of brain death. In: Paradis N, Halperin H, Nowak R (Eds) *Cardiac Arrest. The Science and Practice of Resuscitation Medicine.* Williams & Wilkins, London, p902–20.

Gershlick A, More R (1998) Treatment of myocardial infarction. *British Medical Journal* **316**: 280–4.

Holzer M (2002) The hypothermia after cardiac arrest study group. Mild therapeutic hypothermia to improve neurological outcome after cardiac arrest. *New England Journal of Medicine* **346**:549–56.

International Liaison Committee on Resuscitation (ILCOR) (2003) Therapeutic Hypothermia After Cardiac Arrest: an advisory statement by the Advanced Life Support Task Force of the International Liason Committee on Resuscitation. *Circulation* **108**:118.

Intensive Care Society (2002) *Guidelines for the Transport of Critically Ill Patient.* Intensive Care Society, London.

Jevon P (2006) Chest examination part 2 – chest percussion. *Nursing Times* **102**(45):26–7.

Jevon P, Cunnington A (2006) Chest examination part 3 – chest auscultation. *Nursing Times* **102**(46):26–7.

Jorgensen E (1997) Course of neurological recovery and cerebral prognostic signs during cardiopulmonary resuscitation. *Resuscitation* **35**:9–16.

Kagstrom E, Smith M, Siesjo B (1983) Cerebral circulatory responses to hypercapnia and hyperoxia in the recovery period following complete and incomplete ischaemia in the rat. *Acta Physiologica Scandinavica* **118**:281–91.

Longstreth W, Diehr P, Inui T (1983) Prediction of awakening after out-of-hospital cardiac arrest. *New England Journal of Medicine* **308**:1378–82.

Marik P, Iglesias J (1999) Study NORASEPT 11 Investigators. Low-dose dopamine does not prevent acute renal failure in patients with septic shock and oliguria. *American Journal of Medicine* **197**:387–90.

Minamisawa H, Smith M, Siesjo B (1990) The effect of mild hyperthermia and hypothermia on brain damage following 5, 10 and 15 minutes of forebrain ischaemia. *Annals of Neurology* **28**:26–33.

Mullie A, Verstringe P, Buylaert W *et al.* (1988) Predictive value of Glasgow coma score for awakening after out-of-hospital cardiac arrest. *Lancet* **1**:137–40.

Pulsineli W, Waldman S, Rawlinson D *et al.* (1982) Moderate hyperglycaemia augments ischaemic brain damage: neuropathologic study in the rat. *Neurology* **32**:1239–46.

Resuscitation Council (UK) (2006) *Advanced Life Support*, 5th Ed. Resuscitation Council (UK), London.

Roine R, Kaste M, Kinnunen A *et al.* (1990) Nimodipine after resuscitation from out-of-hospital ventricular fibrillation. A placebo controlled double-blind randomized trial. *Journal of the American Medical Association* **264**:3171–7.

Siesjo B (1978) *Brain Energy Metabolism*. John Wiley & Sons, New York.

Skinner D, Vincent R (1997) *Cardiopulmonary Resuscitation*, 2nd Ed. Oxford University Press, Oxford

Smith G (2003) *ALERT Acute Life-Threatening Events Recognition and Treatment*, 2nd Ed. University of Portsmouth, Portsmouth.

Talley N, O'Connor S (2001) *Clinical Examination: A Systemic Guide to Physical Diagnosis*. Blackwell Publishing, Oxford.

Chapter 14

Bereavement

Introduction

Sudden death, which is recognised as one of the most traumatic events that can be experienced, can leave bereaved relatives struggling to cope with their feelings and reactions. Supporting bereaved relatives is not easy. Healthcare professionals need to know how to help people through the process of grieving. Early correct handling of those who have been suddenly bereaved can greatly ease their journey through the phases of grief and help reduce complications (Resuscitation Council (UK), 2006).

The aim of this chapter is to understand the general principles of managing bereavement. If a more comprehensive and detailed account is required, this can be found elsewhere.

Learning objectives

At the end of this chapter the reader will be able to:

- Describe an ideal layout for the relatives' room
- Discuss the principles of breaking bad news
- Discuss the principles of telephone notification of relatives
- Outline the practical arrangements following a death
- Discuss the issues involved with relatives witnessing resuscitation

Ideal layout for the relatives room

The relatives' room should be spacious, well lit and, if possible, have a window to the outside. This will help to reduce relatives' concerns about being claustrophobic and isolated. In addition, the relatives' room should ideally have the following:

- Comfortable domestic chairs and sofas, including provision for people with special needs
- Telephone with direct dial-in/dial-out facilities and telephone directories
- Wash basin with soap, towel, mirror, freshen-up pack and tissues
- Television/radio available but not prominent
- Hot and cold drinks, fridge, kettle and a non-institutional tea/coffee set
- Books and toys for children
- Access to toilet facilities

Breaking bad news

Who should tell the relatives

If the relatives are not present when the patient dies, or if they arrive after the death, someone will have to break the news to them. When the death is unexpected the most senior doctor available, with a senior nurse in support, should tell the relatives. The doctor is then at hand to answer the inevitable questions concerning the mode of death and what had been done to try and prevent it. In some situations, e.g. when the death is expected, the senior nurse may be the best person to tell the relatives.

Preparation

Adequate preparation is essential. All the relevant information of the deceased, including medical and resuscitation details, should be gathered together. Self-preparation, e.g. washing hands, checking clothing for blood, is also important. The name of the closest relative of the deceased should be sought.

Good communication techniques

- Introduce yourself and colleague(s), confirm they are the correct relatives and identify who is who the closest relative
- Sit down in order to be at the same level of the relatives; establish and maintain eye contact

- Allow time, do not rush and allow periods of silence so that the information can be absorbed
- Avoid platitudes such as 'I know what you are going through', rather reflect back on their emotions, e.g. 'It must be a terrible shock for you'
- Answer questions in a sympathetic and non-judgmental way
- If appropriate, share a cup of tea. This can help the relationship

What to tell the relatives

The way bad news is broken is critical. Words like dead or died are unequivocal and will not be misinterpreted. Honest direct information about the sequence of events, from practitioners who do not skirt around the real issues is valued by relatives.

The use of euphemisms is not recommended (Resuscitation Council (UK), 2006). Although the following phrases may be well meaning, they can lead to a misunderstanding:

- 'She has passed on'
- 'He has slipped away'
- 'She has gone to a better place'
- 'We have lost him'

Telephone notification of relatives

Telephone notification of relatives can be difficult and is never easy. To minimise confusion and misunderstanding, the information should be clear and concise. The following is recommended:

- Identify yourself and the hospital
- Establish who the person is you are speaking to – if this is not the key relative where can he/she be found?
- Give the name of the patient and ward. It seems to be common practice not to inform relatives over the telephone that the patient has died, but instead to tell them that the patient's condition has deteriorated rapidly, is critical, or words to that effect. A dilemma arises if the relatives ask if their loved one

has died. The author's view is that an honest approach is preferable. If the hospital is easily accessible then the relatives can be told when they arrive and not over the phone

- Check that the relatives are clear about the message and are familiar with how to get to the hospital
- Document the exact details of the telephone conversation

Practical arrangements following a death

Cultural and religious requirements: where possible cultural and religious requirements must be respected. Expressions of grief and handling the body can vary depending on the patient's religion and cultural background. Involving the appropriate religious representative can be beneficial.

Viewing the body: being in the presence of their loved one can help relatives work through the grieving process (Resuscitation Council (UK), 2006). They should therefore be given an opportunity to view the body. If the patient has mutilating injuries, encouraging the relatives to view the body may not be advisable.

Legal requirements: the coroner may need to be notified and a post mortem may need to be undertaken to establish the cause of death. Sometimes the coroner may require certain tubes etc. to be left *in situ*. Local policies relating to this will need to be followed.

Information for relatives: the relatives should be provided with the necessary information explaining what to do next. Healthcare organisations usually have helpful literature (Figure 14.1).

General practitioner: the patient's general practitioner will need to be notified.

Primary care agencies: primary care agencies, e.g. social services, may also need to be notified.

Counselling: counselling for the relatives and hospital staff may also be required.

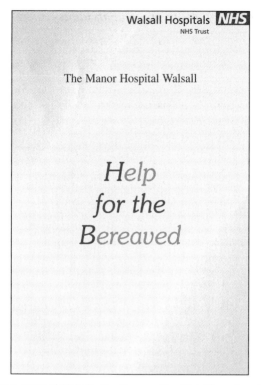

Fig. 14.1 Front cover of *Help for the Bereaved* booklet. Reproduced with permission of Walsall Hospitals NHS Trust.

Relatives witnessing resuscitation

Being separated from a loved one, particularly at the time of death, can cause considerable distress. Should relatives therefore be present during resuscitation?

This issue has been extensively debated in the literature in recent years. Some practitioners believe that relatives should be allowed to witness resuscitation. Others point out that, having relatives present, can cause anxiety for junior doctors, other staff and also for the relatives themselves, particularly if invasive procedures are being undertaken (Resuscitation Council (UK), 2006).

Advantages of relatives witnessing resuscitation

There are a number of advantages with relatives witnessing resuscitation. Being present at the resuscitation:

- Reinforces the fact that their loved one has died, avoiding prolonged denial and assisting with the bereavement process
- Avoids distress that would have been brought on by being separated from their loved one
- Enables the relatives to talk to their loved one when he still may be able to hear them
- Allows the relatives to see for themselves that everything possible was done
- Allows the relatives to touch and speak with the deceased while the body is still warm

(Resuscitation Council (UK), 2006)

Disadvantages of relatives witnessing resuscitation

There are some disadvantages with relatives witnessing resuscitation. Being present at the resuscitation:

- Can cause distress, particularly if invasive procedures are undertaken
- May hinder the cardiac arrest team, physically or emotionally

Necessary safeguards when relatives witness resuscitation

The Resuscitation Council (UK) (2006) recommends that practitioners should identify and respect relatives' wishes to remain with their loved one during resuscitation. However a number of safeguards relating to the relatives being present that must be met. It is important to:

- Notify the members of the crash team of their presence
- Provide a clear explanation of what they will encounter in the resuscitation room
- Allocate a senior member of staff to accompany them and explain the procedures

- Maintain their safety throughout the resuscitation, particularly during defibrillation
- Request that they do not interfere with the resuscitation process
- Ensure they understand that they can leave and return at any time
- Allow them to touch their loved one only when it is safe to do so

Chapter summary

Nurses need to know how to support bereaved relatives through the process of grieving following a patient's death. This chapter has discussed the principles of the early management of bereavement, including how to break bad news. Allowing relatives to witness resuscitation can help with the bereavement process.

Reference

Resuscitation Council (UK) (2006) *Advanced Life Support*, 5th Ed. Resuscitation Council (UK), London.

Chapter 15

Ethical Issues in Resuscitation

Elaine Walton and Phil Jevon

Introduction

The main purpose of medical treatment is to benefit the patient by restoring or maintaining health as far as possible, maximising benefit and minimising harm; if treatment is not beneficial, or if an adult competent patient refuses treatment, the purpose of medical treatment cannot be realised and the justification for providing it is removed (British Medical Association (BMA) *et al.*, 2007a).

Cardiopulmonary resuscitation (CPR) is a form of treatment, which can in theory be undertaken in any patient when cardiac or respiratory function ceases. However, as failure of these functions is inevitable when a patient dies, it is important to identify patients for whom cardiopulmonary arrest represents a terminal event in their illness and in whom CPR is not beneficial and is therefore inappropriate. When CPR is inappropriate, or is indeed against the wishes of a patient with capacity, a do not attempt resuscitation (DNAR) decision should be considered.

Decisions Relating to Cardiopulmonary Resuscitation, the updated joint statement from the British Medical Association (BMA), Resuscitation Council (UK) and the Royal College of Nursing (RCN) (2007), outlines the ethical and legal standards for planning patient care and decision making in relation to CPR.

The nurse has a professional responsibility to ensure that the patient's best interests and well-being are always promoted and safeguarded (Nursing and Midwifery Council (NMC), 2008).

The aim of this chapter is to understand the ethical issues in resuscitation.

Learning outcomes

At the end of the chapter the reader will be able to:

- Outline the ethical principles that guide medical practice
- Discuss the historical background to DNAR decisions
- Discuss the importance of DNAR decisions
- List the key messages in *Decisions Relating to Cardiopulmonary Resuscitation*
- Provide an overview of the DNAR decision-making process
- Outline the factors underpinning DNAR decisions
- Discuss the documentation of DNAR decisions
- Outline DNAR written information requirements for patients and relatives

Ethical principles that guide medical practice

There are two key ethical theories, which guide medical practice. Deontology (duty-based theory), the basic tenet of which is, 'I must always carry out my duty' and utilitarianism (consequence-based theory), which asserts that an action is right if it produces the greatest benefit for the greatest number of people.

In addition, there are four guiding ethical principles which should be used in any decision-making process:

- *Nonmaleficence* – (primum non nocere) first and above all, do no harm
- *Beneficence* – do good, promote good, remove evil or harm
- *Respect for autonomy* – taking into account and acting on the patient's wishes
- *Justice* – fairness, entitlement or right

(Beauchamp & Childress, 2001)

These theories and principles can aid decision making by asking six simple questions:

- What is your duty in this particular circumstance?
- By carrying out my duty, will my actions produce the best available consequences for all concerned?
- Will my actions harm anyone, particularly the patient?

- Am I going to do or promote good for those concerned?
- Am I respecting the patient's wishes?
- Are my actions fair to all concerned?

(Jevon, 2009)

Although this may over-simplify the decision-making process, it does provide a helpful ethical guide. *The Code: Standards of Conduct, Performance and Ethics for Nurses and Midwives* (NMC, 2008) takes these issues into account; so working within the confines of this code will ensure the nurse acts not only within the law but also in a professional and ethical manner.

Historical background to DNAR decisions

Historically, issuing a DNAR decision was considered part of the doctor's 'therapeutic prerogative', and often not formally registered in the patient's records, but 'understood' or 'indicated' by secret markings in the records or on the bed (Holm & Jorgenson, 2001). Such practices may still exist where medical litigation is still uncommon and there are no formal guidelines or policies.

In some situations, discussion and consultation about DNAR decisions had been carried out by staff least experienced or equipped to undertake such sensitive tasks (BMA *et al.*, 1999). In addition, poor communication and documentation in respect of DNAR decisions, could result in CPR being carried out or withheld inappropriately.

Nurses often left DNAR decisions to their medical colleagues; it is perhaps deemed easier to follow medical orders than be the patient's advocate and take on board their values and wishes.

Concerns regarding DNAR decisions

Concerns have been raised regarding DNAR decisions. In 1991, following a case brought to the attention of the Health Service Commissioner regarding a very junior doctor making a DNAR decision, the then Chief Medical Officer wrote to all consultants in England, reiterating their responsibility for ensuring a resuscitation policy was in place and understood by all staff who may be involved, particularly junior medical staff (Chief Medical Officer, 1991).

The much publicised case of Kathryn Knight in 2000, a 67-year-old lady with an inoperable gastric carcinoma, highlighted concerns regarded DNAR decisions (Baker, 2000). She had been admitted to hospital with septicaemia (probably a complication of chemotherapy). A junior doctor, who had never seen or consulted Ms Knight, documented in her notes 'in view of the diagnosis, in the event of a cardiac arrest it would be inappropriate to resuscitate'. To make matters worse Ms Knight was not informed of the decision. She only found out by chance about it during an out-patients department consultation.

In April 2000, Age Concern issued a press release stating that some doctors were ignoring national guidelines on the resuscitation of older people and that older people had found 'not for resuscitation' recorded in their medical notes without their agreement or knowledge (Luttrell, 2001). This lead to Professor Shah Ebrahim publishing an editorial in the *British Medical Journal* (BMJ) stating that doctors regularly issue 'Do Not Resuscitate' orders for patients without their knowledge; he claimed that black people, alcohol misusers, non-English speakers and those with human immunodeficiency virus (HIV) are more likely to get a DNAR order, suggesting that prejudice is influencing medical decisions (Ebrahim, 2000).

This combination of events was followed by intense media interest and concern regarding how DNAR decisions were being made. Such was the level of concern that the NHS Executive issued a Health Service Circular to all National Health Service (NHS) Trust Chief Executives in September 2000 stipulating that appropriate resuscitation policies should be in place which respected patients' rights, were understood by all relevant staff and were subject to appropriate audit and monitoring (NHS Executive, 2000).

Media interest in DNAR decisions remains. The Daily Mail in its report *Hospital gave order to let our mother die, say sisters* it states that 'an elderly woman was left to die in hospital after an order not to resuscitate her was issued without her family's knowledge' (Daily Mail, 2008).

BMA, Resuscitation Council UK and RCN guidelines

To improve DNAR decision-making, the BMA, Resuscitation Council (UK) and the RCN have produced guidelines on how and when DNAR decisions should be considered. First published in 1993 (BMA *et al.*, 1993), these guidelines have been subsequently revised and updated (BMA *et al.*, 1999, 2001); the latest guidelines *Decisions Relating to cardiopulmonary resuscitation* were published in October 2007 and take into account the Mental Capacity Act 2005 (BMA *et al.*, 2007a).

The guidelines provide a framework to:

- Support decisions relating to CPR
- Ensure effective communication
- Provide the general principals that allow for CPR policies to be tailored to local circumstances

(BMA *et al.*, 2007a)

Local policies may then provide further, more detailed guidance, for example related to information about individual responsibilities (BMA *et al.*, 2007a).

All healthcare organizations/providers that have to make decisions about resuscitation, e.g. hospitals, GP surgeries, care homes and ambulance services, should have a resuscitation policy which includes DNAR decisions (BMA *et al.*, 2007a); this policy should be readily available and understood by all relevant staff (NHS Executive, 2000).

Importance of DNAR decisions

Kouwenhoven and his colleagues first described closed-chest cardiac massage in the 1960s (Kouwenhoven *et al.*, 1960). They commented 'Anyone, anywhere, can now initiate cardiac resuscitative procedures. All that is needed are two hands.'

However, although modern resuscitation techniques have resulted in the successful resuscitation of many patients, they unfortunately have also made it possible to bring 'dead' patients back to life, prolong the process of dying and deny patients dignified and peaceful deaths with their loved ones present (Baskett *et al.*, 2005). 'You can treat and must not kill, but do not try to bring a dead soul back to life' (Pinder, fifth century BC cited in Negovsky, 1993).

It has been shown that, following a cardiac arrest in hospital, 50% of patients do not even survive the CPR attempt

(Tunstall-Pedoe *et al.*, 1992; Holland *et al.*, 1998), while less than 20% survive to discharge (Tunstall-Pedoe *et al.*, 1992). In 25% of CPR attempts, the process of dying is merely being prolonged (Snowden *et al.*, 1984). Resuscitation attempts are unsuccessful in 70–95% of cases and death is ultimately inevitable (Baskett *et al.*, 2005).

A valid DNAR decision is therefore important to prevent unnecessary CPR.

Key messages in *Decisions Relating to Cardiopulmonary Resuscitation*

The key messages in *Decisions Relating to Cardiopulmonary Resuscitation* are:

- Decisions about CPR should be made following an individual assessment of the patient's case
- Advance care planning, which should include decisions relating to CPR, is an important aspect of sound clinical management of patients at risk of cardiorespiratory arrest
- Communication and the provision of information are essential parts of effective quality care
- Discussion about CPR is not necessary if the patient is unlikely to suffer a cardiorespiratory arrest
- If no explicit decision has been made in advance, there should be initial presumption in favour of CPR
- If CPR would not re-start the heart and breathing, it shouldn't be attempted
- If the anticipated benefits of performing CPR could be outweighed by the burdens, the patient's informed views are of paramount importance; if the patient lacks capacity, those close to him should be included in discussions to try to establish his wishes, feelings, beliefs and values
- If a patient with capacity refuses CPR, or a patient lacking capacity has a valid and applicable advance decision refusing CPR, his wishes should be respected
- A DNAR order decision does not override clinical judgment in the rare event when the cardiac arrest has a reversible cause that does not match the circumstances envisaged

- A DNAR decision applies only to CPR, not to any other aspects of treatment

(BMA *et al.*, 2007a)

Overview of the DNAR decision-making process

The flowchart in Figure 15.1 provides an overview of the DNAR decision-making process. The very helpful flowchart provides clear guidance to the procedures that should be followed when considering a DNAR decision.

Factors underpinning DNAR decisions

Importance of advance care planning

The risk of cardiopulmonary arrest is low in the majority of patients who receive healthcare in the hospital and community setting; there is no ethical or legal requirement to discuss every possible eventuality with the patient; if the risk of cardiopulmonary arrest is considered to be low, then it is not necessary to initiate discussion about CPR (BMA *et al.*, 2007a).

However, there are patients who will be identified at risk of cardiopulmonary arrest, such as those with an incurable underlying condition (e.g. cancer), severe acute illness (e.g. stroke) or at the end of life stage, for whom it would be desirable to make decisions about CPR (BMA *et al.*, 2007a). Appropriate advanced care planning should be considered an essential component in good clinical practice.

Justification for treatment

The aim of healthcare is to benefit the patient, by restoring/ maintaining his health, maximising benefit and minimising harm; treatment can no longer be justified if it fails or ceases to be beneficial, or if an adult patient with capacity refuses treatment (BMA *et al.*, 2007a).

Although prolonging life can be beneficial, it is not appropriate to do so at all costs with no regard to quality of life or to the potential burdens the treatment ('successful CPR') will bring to

DO NOT ATTEMPT RESUSCITATION (DNAR) ORDER

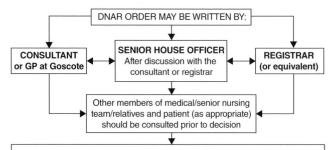

DNAR ORDER MAY BE WRITTEN BY:

| CONSULTANT or GP at Goscote | **SENIOR HOUSE OFFICER** After discussion with the consultant or registrar | **REGISTRAR** (or equivalent) |

Other members of medical/senior nursing team/relatives and patient (as appropriate) should be consulted prior to decision

DOCUMENTATION

- **'Not For Attempted Cardiopulmonary Resuscitation'** should be documented legibly in the medical and nursing notes along with the date and time of the order being made
- If written by the SHO, the name of the consultant or registrar who has agreed the DNAR order should be documented in the medical notes
- Reason for the order and any discussions undertaken with the patient or relatives should be documented. If it is inappropriate to discuss the decision with either patient and /or relatives, the reason for this should be clearly documented
- If specific review times are inappropriate the reasons for this should be documented along with the next review time, Also, the name of the consultant or registrar who has agreed to different review times should be recorded if written by the SHO

COMMUNICATION
Ensure that the decision is communicated to:
- Other relevant health professionals
- Relatives and patients as appropriate

REVIEW
The DNAR order should be reviewed and re-recorded:
- **Within 72 hours** at the Manor
- **With 1 week** at Goscote
- **On transfer** to the care of another consultant, or hospital
- **At the discretion of the consultant or registrar involved wth the order (refer to documentation box)**

DNAR ORDER APPLIES UNTIL IT IS REVIEWED
and RE-CONFIRMED, AND FOR THE DURATION
OF THAT HOSPITAL ADMISSION ONLY

Fig. 15.1 Flowchart outlining the 'do not attempt resuscitation' decision-making process. Reproduced with permission of Walsall Hospitals NHS Trust.

the patient; the decision to undertake CPR should be based on the balance of burdens, risks and benefits to the patient (BMA *et al.*, 2007a).

Non-discrimination

Any CPR decision made should be individualized to the patient's particular circumstances and should not be influenced by age, disability or a healthcare professional's personal view of the patient's quality of life; a blanket policy that denies CPR to a particular group of patients (e.g. all patients in a hospice) is considered unethical and probably unlawful (BMA *et al.*, 2007a).

Human Rights Act 1998

The Human Rights Act 1998 incorporates the majority of the rights set out in the European Convention on Human Rights into UK law. In order to meet their obligations under the Act, health professionals must be able to demonstrate that their decisions are compatible with the human rights identified in the Articles of the Convention (Resuscitation Council (UK), 2006). Provisions particularly relevant to DNAR orders include the right to:

- Life (Article 2)
- Be free from inhuman or degrading treatment (Article 3)
- Respect for privacy and family life (Article 8)
- Freedom of expression (Article 10)
- Be free from discriminatory practices in respect of these rights (Article 14)

(BMA *et al.*, 2007a)

Presumptions in favour of CPR

In the absence of a valid DNAR decision, CPR should be commenced in the event of the patient having a cardiorespiratory arrest.

However, if CPR is inappropriate, e.g. for a patient who is in the final stages of a terminal illness, where death is imminent and CPR would be unsuccessful, it should not be started even in the absence of a DNAR decision; a nurse who makes a considered decision not to start CPR should be supported by colleagues and her employer (BMA *et al.*, 2007a).

Mental Health Act 2005 and Adults with Incapacity Act 2000

The Mental Health Act 2005 (England & Wales) and the Adults with Incapacity Act 2000 (Scotland), provide guidance concerning proxy decision makers and their role when the patient lacks decision-making capacity (lacks capacity).

Liverpool Care Pathway

The Liverpool Care Pathway (LCP), which is currently being implemented across the UK, provides a comprehensive evidence-based template for multi-disciplinary care for last few days of life; Goal 3 of the initial assessment specifically reminds the clinician to consider and document the patient's CPR status (BMA *et al.*, 2007a).

Who can make a DNAR decision

The overall responsibility for making a DNAR decision rests with the most senior clinician in charge of the patient's care as defined by the local DNAR policy (it may be delegated to another competent person) (BMA *et al.*, 2007a); in most situations this will be a registered medical practitioner but in some situations, such as in nurse-led palliative care services, a senior nurse with appropriate training may fulfill this role, subject to local discussion and agreement (BMA *et al.*, 2007b).

A DNAR decision should ideally be agreed with other appropriate members of the healthcare team (BMA *et al.*, 2007a); if there is genuine doubt or disagreement about whether CPR would be clinically appropriate a further senior clinical opinion should be sought (BMA *et al.*, 2007b).

However, the nurse must always act always in such a manner as to promote and safeguard the interests and well-being of the patient and should recognise and respect the uniqueness and dignity of each patient (NMC, 2008). If the nurse is of the opinion that CPR is not appropriate for a patient, or is indeed aware that the patient does not wish to be resuscitated in the event of a cardiac arrest, then she should raise the issue with senior medical colleagues at the earliest opportunity. In some situations, as described above, the senior nurse will be making the DNAR decision (BMA *et al.*, 2007a).

DNAR decision based on clinical grounds

In some cases a DNAR decision is made on clinical grounds, i.e. CPR will not be successful at restarting breathing and circulation; in these situations, it is not necessary or appropriate to ascertain the patient's wishes regarding CPR, unless he has expressed a specific wish to do so (BMA *et al.*, 2007a). It is usual practice to inform the relatives of the decision.

DNAR decision based on benefits and burdens

A DNAR decision based on balancing benefits and burdens of CPR should take into account the:

- Likely clinical outcome and level of realistic recovery
- Patient's own or ascertainable wishes, views, feelings, beliefs and values
- Patient's human rights (see above)
- Likelihood of the patient experiencing severe unmanageable pain or suffering
- Level of the patient's awareness of his existence and surroundings

(BMA *et al.*, 2007a)

Should the patient be consulted?

The rights of the patient are central to decision making on resuscitation. Patients have as much right to be involved in DNAR decisions as they do with other decisions about their care and treatment (Department of Health, 2000). In fact, approximately 90% of patients would prefer to discuss the issue of CPR and there are often inconsistencies between what the patient wants and what the medical staff think the patient wants (Broekman, 1998). When a DNAR decision is based on considerations related to established benefits and burdens, the views of the patient should be sought (BMA *et al.*, 2007a).

However, when a DNAR decision is made on clinical grounds, i.e. CPR will not be successful at restarting breathing and circulation, it is unnecessary and inappropriate to explore the patient's wishes regarding CPR, unless he has expressed a specific wish to do so (BMA *et al.*, 2007a).

Patient with capacity

If a patient with capacity (mental power) is at risk of cardiac or respiratory arrest, and the healthcare team is doubtful whether the benefits of undertaking CPR will outweigh the burdens and whether the predicted post-successful recovery will be acceptable for the patient, sensitive exploration of the patient's wishes, feelings, beliefs and values should be sought (BMA *et al.*, 2007a). Any discussions with the patient should be accurately documented.

Clinicians who discuss or communicate DNAR decisions with patients should:

- Provide patients with as much information as they wish
- Provide information in such a manner and format that patients can understand it (an interpreter may be required)
- Answer questions a honestly as possible
- Explain the aims of treatment.

(BMA *et al.*, 2007a)

If a patient does not accept a DNAR decision which has been made on clinical grounds, then careful explanation of the reasons for the decision is required; if requested, a second opinion should be arranged wherever possible (the same procedure applies to relatives should they disagree with a DNAR decision) (BMA *et al.*, 2007a).

Patient who lacks capacity

If a patient, who lacks capacity, is at risk of cardiac or respiratory arrest, and the healthcare team is doubtful whether the benefits of undertaking CPR will outweigh the burdens, discussions should take place within the healthcare team about a DNAR decision (BMA *et al.*, 2007a). The patient's best interests must be central to the decision-making process.

Relatives

Those close to the patient should be consulted; this is considered good practice and is probably a requirement of the Human Rights

Act 1998 (Article 8 – right to private and family life; Article 10 – right to impart and receive information) and the Mental Capacity Act 2005 (BMA *et al.*, 2007a). It must be emphasised that those close to the patient have no legal authority in the decision-making process and that their role is purely to help the clinician in the decision-making process.

Lasting power of attorney

The Mental Capacity Act 2005 (England & Wales) allows an adult, who has capacity, to make a lasting power of attorney (LPA), appointing someone to make decisions about his healthcare (welfare attorney), should he ever lack the capacity to make them himself (BMA *et al.*, 2007a). An attorney is a person, especially a lawyer, appointed to act for another in business or legal matters (Thompson, 1998).

However, before relying on the authority of the welfare attorney, the healthcare team should be satisfied that:

- The patient lacks capacity to make a DNAR decision
- A statement has been included in the LPA, stipulating that the welfare attorney can make decisions about life-prolonging treatment
- The LPA has been registered with the Office of the Public Guardian
- The decision made by the welfare attorney is in the best interests of the patient

(BMA *et al.*, 2007a)

If CPR is clinically inappropriate, the welfare attorney cannot demand that it is carried out. However, if CPR is likely to restart the heart and the DNAR decision is to be based on the balance between benefits and burdens, the welfare attorney should be consulted concerning the patient's likely wishes; if there is a disagreement which can not be resolved through discussion and a second clinical opinion, the court of protection may be asked to make a declaration (BMA *et al.*, 2007a).

Mental capacity advocate

The Mental Capacity Act 2005 stipulates that an independent mental capacity advocate (IMCA) should be consulted concerning all decisions about serious medical treatment, where the patient lacks capacity and there is no one, e.g. a relative or welfare attorney, able to speak on his behalf. Where there is genuine doubt whether CPR would be successful or if a DNAR decision is being considered on the balance of benefits and burdens, an IMCA must be involved (BMA *et al.*, 2007a). If a DNAR decision is being considered, but an IMCA is not available (e.g. at night or at a weekend), it should be discussed with the IMCA at the earliest opportunity (BMA *et al.*, 2007a).

Advance decisions

An advance decision (formally referred to as advance directive or living will) is related to end-of-life treatment. It should be in writing, and as long as it is valid and applicable, should be followed and treatment not provided. It takes precedence over any view that anyone else may have about what is in the best interests of the person in question, even if the result is that the decision results in the person dying.

When to ignore or suspend a DNAR decision

Occasionally a patient with a DNAR decision may suffer a cardiac or respiratory arrest caused by a readily reversible cause, e.g. choking on a foreign body, anaphylaxis. In these rare situations, unless the patient has specifically refused intervention, it would be appropriate to initiate CPR (BMA *et al.*, 2007a).

Similarly, it may be appropriate to suspend a DNAR decision if the patient is is undertaking a procedure which carries a risk of a potentially reversible cardiac arrest, e.g. cardiac catheterization (ventricular fibrillation) (BMA *et al.*, 2007a).

Documentation of DNAR decisions

Any discussions with the patient, relatives and healthcare team about DNAR decisions should be documented, signed and dated in the patient's health records. It should also be documented if the patient has stated he does not wish to be involved in such discussions.

To avoid confusion, it is recommended to use the phrase '*Do Not Attempt Cardiopulmonary Resuscitation*' when documenting a

DNAR decision (BMA *et al.*, 2007a). In addition, other pertinent information should be documented following local guidelines including:

- Date and time decision was made
- Who made the decision
- Rationale
- Discussions with patient, relatives and healthcare team
- Review date/time

DNAR decisions should be reviewed on a regular basis, which should be determined by the clinician in charge and will be influenced by the clinical circumstances of the patient. Local policies should include safeguards to ensure that a review occurs appropriately, and that the patient's ability to participate in the decision-making process may change depending on his clinical condition. However, it is generally not necessary to discuss the DNAR decision with the patient each time it is reviewed, unless the decision is changed (BMA *et al.*, 2007a).

Some healthcare establishments have devised DNAR forms which are intended to assist the clinician with making a DNAR decision. These have been seen improve the clarity of the DNAR statement, particularly by whom, when it has been documented, and the reasons for the decision (Castle *et al.*, 2003; Diggory *et al.*, 2003, 2004; Cauchi *et al.*, 2004; Harris & Linnane, 2005). The Resuscitation Council (UK) is currently in the process of developing a model DNAR form that individual establishments may wish to adopt.

Information for patients and relatives

The BMA's Ethics Department has issued a model patient leaflet *Decisions Relating to Cardiopulmonary Resuscitation* (BMA, 2008) (Figure 15.2). It provides the patient with information to assist him in making decisions related to his treatment and may be useful to relatives, friends and carers. It states what CPR is and whether it is relevant to consider issues related to this, and how decisions are made about whether it should be attempted or not. This model information leaflet can be amended to include local information and can be obtained from the BMA's website (http://

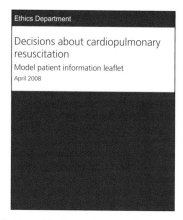

Fig. 15.2 DNAR leaflet to guide the decision-making process.

www.bma.org.uk/ethics/cardiopulmonary_resuscitation/
CPRpatientinformation.jsp).

Such information should be readily available to all patients and people close to the patient, and written information about CPR policies should be included in the general literature provided to patients about healthcare organisations. In addition, the DNAR policy should be readily available to those who may wish to consult it, including patients, relatives and carers (Department of Health, 2000).

Chapter summary

In this chapter an overview to ethical issues in resuscitation has been provided. The historical background to DNAR decisions and their importance have been discussed. The key messages in *Decisions Relating to Cardiopulmonary Resuscitation* have been listed and an overview of the DNAR decision-making process has been provided. The factors underpinning DNAR decisions have been highlighted, together with documentation issues and written information requirements for patients and relatives.

Further information
Medical Ethics Department
British Medical Association
BMA House
Tavistock Square

London WC1H 9JP
Tel 020 7383 6286

Resuscitation Council (UK)
5th Floor, Tavistock House North
Tavistock Square
London WC1H 9HR
Tel 020 7388 4678

Royal College of Nursing
20 Cavendish Square
London W1 0AB
Tel 020 7409 3333

References

Age Concern (2000) *Not for Resuscitation Your Life in Their Hands.* Age Concern, London.

Baskett P, Steen P, Bossaert L (2005) European Resuscitation Council Guidelines for Resuscitation 2005 Section 8. The ethics of resuscitation and end-of-life decisions. *Resuscitation* S171–S180.

Baker J (2000) Doctors were told to just to let me die. *Daily Express*, 14 April.

Beauchamp TL, Childress JF (2001) *Principles of Biomedical Ethics*, 5th Ed. Oxford University Press, Oxford.

British Medical Association, Resuscitation Council (UK), Royal College of Nursing (1993) *Decisions Relating to Cardiopulmonary Resuscitation. A joint statement from the British Medical Association, the Resuscitation Council (UK) and the Royal College of Nursing.* BMA, London.

British Medical Association, Resuscitation Council (UK), Royal College of Nursing (1999) *Decisions Relating to Cardiopulmonary Resuscitation. A joint statement from the British Medical Association, the Resuscitation Council (UK) and the Royal College of Nursing.* BMA, London.

British Medical Association, Resuscitation Council (UK), Royal College of Nursing (2001) *Decisions Relating to Cardiopulmonary Resuscitation. A joint statement from the British Medical Association, the Resuscitation Council (UK) and the Royal College of Nursing.* BMA, London.

British Medical Association, Resuscitation Council (UK), Royal College of Nursing (2007a) *Decisions Relating to Cardiopulmonary Resuscitation. A Joint Statement from the British Medical Association, the Resuscitation Council (U)K and the Royal College of Nursing.* BMA, London.

BMA, Resuscitation Council (UK), Royal College of Nursing (2007b) *Decisions Relating to Cardiopulmonary Resuscitation. A Joint Statement from the British Medical Association, the Resuscitation Council (U)K and the Royal College of Nursing.* BMA, London – updated November 2007.

British Medical Association (2008) *Decisions about Cardiopulmonary Resuscitation: Model Patient Leaflet.* BMA, London.

Broekman B (1998) Discussing resuscitation with patients, why not? *Resuscitation* **37**:2062.

Castle N, Owen R, Kenwood G, Ineson N (2003) Pre-printed 'Do Not Attempt Resuscitation' forms improve documentation? *Resuscitation* **59**:85–95.

Cauchi L, Vigus J, Diggory P (2004) Implementation of cardiopulmonary resuscitation in elderly care departments across: a survey of 13 hospitals shows wide variability in practice. *Resuscitation* **63**:157–60.

Chief Medical Officer (1991) *(PL/CMO(91)22)*. Department of Health, London.

Daily Mail (2008) Hospital gave order to let our mother die, say sisters. *Daily Mail*, Tuesday 25 March, p32.

Department of Health (2000) *Health Service Circular: Resuscitation Policy*. Department of Health, London.

Diggory P, Cauchi L, Griffith D *et al.* (2003) The influence of new guidelines on cardiopulmonary resuscitation (CPR) decisions. Five cycles of audit of a clerk proforma which included a resuscitation decision. *Resuscitation* **56**:159–65.

Diggory P, Shire L, Griffith D *et al.* (2004) Influence of guidelines on cardiopulmonary resuscitation (CPR) decisions: an audit of clerking proforma. *Clinical Medicine* **4**:424–6.

Ebrahim, S. (2000) Do not resuscitate decisions flogging dead horses or a dignified death? *British Medical Journal* **320**:1155–6.

Harris DG, Linnane SJ (2005) Making do not attempt resuscitation decisions: do doctors follow the guidelines? *Hospital Medicine* **66**(1):43–5.

Holland M, Hawkins J, Gill M *et al.* (1998) One year prospective audit of outcome following cardiopulmonary resuscitation on an in-hospital patient population. *Resuscitation* **37**(2):1–3.

Holm S, Jorgenson EO (2001) Ethical issues in cardiopulmonary resuscitation. *Resuscitation* **50**:135–9.

Jevon P (2009) *Care of the dying and deceased patient*. Wiley-Blackwell Publishing, Oxford.

Kouwenhoven W, Jude J, Knickerbocker G (1960) Closed-chest cardiac massage. *Journal of the American Medical Association* **173**:1064–67.

Luttrell, S. (2001) Decisions relating to cardiopulmonary resuscitation: commentary 2: Some concerns. *Journal of Medical Ethics* **27**:321–2.

NHS Executive (2000) *Resuscitation Policy (HSC 2000/028)*. Department of Health, London.

Nursing and Midwifery Council (NMC) (2008) *The Code: Standards of conduct, performance and ethics for nurses and midwives*. NMC, London.

Negovsky VA (1993) Death, dying and revival: ethical aspects. *Resuscitation* **25**:99–107.

Resuscitation Council UK (2006) *Advanced life support*. 5th Ed. Resuscitation Council UK, London.

Snowden G, Baskett P, Robins D (1984) Factors associated with survival and eventual cerebral status following cardiac arrest. *Anaesthesia* **39**:1.

Thompson D (1998) *The Concise Oxford Dictionary*, 9th Ed, Clarendon Press, Oxford.

Tunstall-Pedoe H, Bailey L, Chamberlain D *et al.* (1992) Survey of 3765 cardiopulmonary resuscitations in British Hospitals. The BRESUS Study: methods and overall results. *British Medical Journal* **304**:1347–51.

Chapter 16

Resuscitation Records

Introduction

Maintaining accurate records is an important aspect of nursing (Nursing and Midwifery Council (NMC), 2005, 2008), particularly following a resuscitation attempt. Both the NMC and the Clinical Negligence Scheme for Trusts (CNST) require their members to maintain high standards of record keeping (Dimond, 2005; NMC, 2008).

The aim of this chapter is to understand the principles of maintaining accurate resuscitation records.

Learning outcomes

At the end of the chapter the reader will be able to:

- Discuss why maintaining accurate resuscitation records is important
- List some examples of poor record keeping
- List the factors underpinning effective record keeping
- Outline the importance of auditing records
- Discuss the legal issues associated with record keeping

Why maintaining accurate resuscitation records is important

> *Record keeping is an integral part of nursing, midwifery and health visiting practice. It is a tool of professional practice and one that should help the care process. It is not separate from this process and it is not an optional extra to be fitted in if circumstances allow.*
>
> (NMC, 2005)

An accurate record of the resuscitation attempt will help to protect the welfare of both the patient and the nurses by promoting:

- High standards of clinical and nursing care
- Continuity of patient care
- Effective communication and dissemination of information between members of the inter-professional healthcare team
- An accurate account of treatment and care planning and delivery

The quality of record keeping is also a reflection on the standard of nursing practice: good record keeping is an indication that the practitioner is professional and skilled while poor record keeping often highlights wider problems with the individual's practice (NMC, 2005).

Examples of poor record keeping

Nearly every report published by the Health Service Commissioner (Health Service Ombudsman) following a complaint identifies examples of poor record keeping that have either hampered the care the patient has received or have made it difficult for healthcare professionals to defend their practice (Dimond, 2005).

Examples of poor record keeping encountered include:

- Absence of clarity
- Failure to record action taken when a problem has been identified
- Missing information
- Spelling mistakes
- Inaccurate records

(Dimond, 2005)

Factors underpinning effective record keeping

There is a number of factors that underpin good record keeping. The patient's records should:

- Be factual, consistent and accurate
- Be updated as soon as possible after any recordable event
- Provide current information on the care and condition of the patient
- Be documented clearly and in such a way that the text can not be erased
- Be consecutive and accurately dated, timed and signed (including a printed signature)
- Have any alterations and additions dated, timed and signed; all original entries should be clearly legible
- Not include abbreviations, jargon, meaningless phrases, irrelevant speculation and offensive subjective statements
- Still be legible if photocopied
- Identify any problems identified and most importantly the action taken to rectify them

It is important to record all aspects of patient monitoring. Some observations will be recorded on the patient's observation charts (e.g. the ICU Observation Chart and the Standard Observation Chart). Dates and times should be clearly visible and standard coloured ink should be used, following local protocols. It is also important to ensure that an accurate record is made in the patient's notes. In particular, it is important to include interventions and any response to the interventions.

Best practice – record keeping

Records must be:

- Factual
- Legible
- Clear
- Concise
- Accurate
- Signed
- Timed
- Dated

(Drew *et al.*, 2000)

Importance of auditing resuscitation records

Audit can play an important role in ensuring a quality resuscitation service. In particular, it can help to improve the process of record keeping. By auditing records the standard can be evaluated and any areas for improvement and staff development identified. Audit tools should be developed at a local level to monitor the standards of record keeping.

Audit should primarily be aimed at serving the interests of the patient rather than the organisation (NMC, 2005). A system of peer review may also be of value. Whatever audit system is used, the confidentiality of patients' information applies to audit just as it does to record keeping.

Legal issues associated with record keeping

The patient's records are occasionally required as evidence before a court of law, by the Health Service Commissioner or in order to investigate a complaint at a local level. Sometimes they may be requested by the NMC's Fitness to Practice committees when investigating complaints related to misconduct. Care plans, diaries and anything that makes reference to the patient's care may be required as evidence (NMC, 2005).

What constitutes a legal document is often a cause for concern. Any document requested by the court becomes a legal document (Dimond, 1994), e.g. nursing records, medical records, radiographs, laboratory reports, observation charts; in fact any document which may be relevant to the case.

If any of the documents are missing, the writer of the records may be cross-examined as to the circumstances of their disappearance (Dimond 1994):

> *Medical records are not proof of the truth of the facts stated in them but the maker of the records may be called to give evidence as to the truth as to what is contained in them.*

(Dimond 1994)

The approach to record keeping which courts of law adopt tends to be that if it is not recorded, it has not been undertaken (NMC, 2005). Professional judgment is required when deciding what is relevant and what needs to be recorded, particularly if the patient's clinical condition is apparently unchanging and no record has been made of the care that has been delivered.

A registered nurse has both a professional and a legal duty of care. Consequently when keeping records it is important to be able to demonstrate that:

- A comprehensive nursing assessment of the patient has been undertaken, including care that has been planned and provided
- Relevant information is included together with any measures that have been taken in response to changes in the patient's condition
- The duty of care owed to the patient has been honoured and that no acts or omissions have compromised the patient's safety
- Arrangements have been made for ongoing care of the patient

The registered nurse is also accountable for any delegation of record keeping to members of the multi-professional team who are not registered practitioners. For example, if record keeping is delegated to a pre-registration student nurse or a healthcare assistant, competence to perform the task must be ensured and adequate supervision provided. All such entries must be countersigned.

The Access to Health Records Act 1990 gives patients the right of access to their manually maintained health records which were made after 1st November 1991. The Data Protection Act 1998 gives patients the right to access their computer-held records. The Freedom of Information Act 2000 grants the rights to anyone to all information that is not covered by the Data Protection Act 1998 (NMC, 2005).

Sometimes it is necessary to withhold information, if it could affect the physical or mental well-being of the patient or if it would breach another patient's confidentiality (NMC, 2005). If the decision to withhold information is made, justification for doing so must be clearly recorded in the patient's notes.

Audit and reporting standards

The Royal College of Anaesthetists *et al.* (2008) recommend that the following should be audited to help ensure a high quality resuscitation service:

- The availability and use of resuscitation equipment
- The availability of cardiopulmonary arrest and peri-arrest drugs
- All cardiopulmonary arrests using the principles of the Utstein template
- Do not attempt resuscitation (DNAR) decisions (the audit of DNAR policies is mandatory (NHS Executive, 2000))
- Cardiopulmonary arrest outcomes
- Critical incidents leading to cardiopulmonary arrest or occurring during the resuscitation attempt
- Health and safety issues during resuscitation, e.g. manual handling

Chapter summary

Following resuscitation, it is important to ensure good record keeping. Good record keeping is both the product of good teamwork and an important tool in promoting high-quality healthcare.

References

Dimond, B. (1994) *Legal Aspects in Midwifery*. Midwifery Press, Cheshire.

Dimond B (2005) Exploring common deficiencies that occur in record keeping. *British Journal of Nursing* **14**(10):568–70.

Drew D, Jevon P, Raby M (2000) *Resuscitation of the Newborn*. Butterworth Heinemann, Oxford.

NHS Executive (2000) *Resuscitation Policy* (HSC 2000/028). Department of Health: London.

Nursing and Midwifery Council (2005) *Guidelines for Records and Record Keeping*. NMC, London.

Nursing and Midwifery Council (2008) *The Code: Standards of Conduct, Performance and Ethics for Nurses and Midwives*. NMC, London.

Royal College of Anaesthetists, Royal College of Physicians of London, Intensive Care Society, Resuscitation Council (UK) (2008) *Cardiopulmonary Resuscitation: Standards for Clinical Practice and Training. A Joint Statement from The Royal College of Anaesthetists, The Royal College of Physicians of London, The Intensive Care Society, The Resuscitation Council (UK)*. The Royal College of Anaesthetists, London.

Chapter 17

Resuscitation Training

I hear and I forget, I see and I remember, I do and I understand.
Chinese Proverb

Introduction

The aim of resuscitation training is to equip the learner with the necessary knowledge and skills to perform cardiopulmonary resuscitation (CPR) at a level at which they would be expected to perform, whether they are a lay rescuer, first responder or member of the cardiac arrest team (Baskett *et al.*, 2005).

CPR employs skills that are essentially practical and practitioners need hands-on practical training to both acquire and maintain them. The methods used to teach CPR techniques have been the subject of much investigation in recent years. Considerable effort has been devoted by teachers and educationalists into determining the optimum method of teaching CPR techniques so that the necessary skills are both acquired and easily retained.

The aim of this chapter is to understand the principles of resuscitation training.

Learning outcomes

At the end of the chapter the reader will be able to:

- Discuss why resuscitation training is important
- Outline the principles of adult learning
- Describe the methods of resuscitation training
- List the recommendations for resuscitation training for healthcare staff
- Describe what training mannequins and models are currently available for resuscitation training

Why resuscitation training is important

Resuscitation training is important because:

- Practitioners' skills in resuscitation are often very poor (Lowenstein *et al.*, 1981; Wynne *et al.*, 1987; Buss *et al.*, 1993)
- There is considerable disparity between perceived competence and the actual ability to undertake effective resuscitation (Smith & Hatchett, 1992)
- The experience of senior practitioners attending cardiac arrests is that confidence levels are often high but this is generally not matched by high skill levels (Wynne *et al.*, 1987).
- Retention of CPR skills is very poor (McKenna & Glendon, 1985, Moser & Coleman, 1992; Baskett *et al.*, 2005); significant deterioration in competence has been shown after only 10 weeks (Broomfield, 1996). At present there is unfortunately no consensus on the best way to overcome this problem nor on how often refresher training is required. Certainly the more frequent the updates the better, though realistically an annual one is probably the most achievable

Principles of adult learning

Adults are usually well motivated to learn once they realise that the course content is relevant to them. Adults generally learn best when they are treated as adults and when their skills, experience and prior knowledge are recognised and utilised.

The teacher can facilitate adult learning in several ways:

- Acting as a resource person and helper
- Explaining points that have not been understood
- Demonstrating principles, concepts and skills
- Challenging the learner's values when appropriate
- Adopting the role as task masker and evaluator
- Encouraging learner self-evaluation
- Managing groups of learners effectively and facilitating the pursuit of intellectual questions

(Fuszard, 1995)

Considerable research has been undertaken evaluating the principles of teaching basic and advanced CPR skills and factors affecting their retention. Both course content and time devoted to practice on mannequins will influence skill attainment and subsequent retention of skills.

Constructive feedback during training is important and should not only identify the student's strong points, which will increase the students' confidence and motivation, but should also identify any weaknesses or deficiencies which need to be addressed and require more practice. In the event of poor performance, students should not be ridiculed.

Poor learner motivation, poor student–teacher relationship, physical and environmental factors all can create barriers to adult learning (Rogers, 1986).

Resuscitation training methods

There are various methods of providing resuscitation training. The methods chosen will depend on a number of factors, including time allocation, number of instructors, number of students, equipment, facilities and learning objectives. Quite often a variety of methods is used in each training session.

Regardless of the method used, it is recommended to adopt the following three-part approach to facilitate the teaching and learning process:

- *Set*: ensure the environment (lighting, heating, seating arrangements, audio-visual aids, training mannequins etc.) is adequate for training, set the mood, enhance the learners' motivation, state the session objectives and clarify the roles of the teacher and learners
- *Dialogue* (main teaching part of the session): ensure the content is presented in a clear and logical format and at a level which the learners can understand; answer learners' questions appropriately and check learners have understood the content
- *Closure*: include time for questions and queries from the learners, provide a concise summary and clearly terminate the session

(Resuscitation Council (UK), 2001)

There are four key teaching methods, which can be used in CPR training:

- Lectures
- Skill stations
- Cardiac arrest scenarios
- Discussion groups

Lectures

Lectures can be used to revise core material, highlight key points and complement practical stations, but should not replace practical teaching on mannequins and models. They also provide a valuable opportunity for group discussion. To help maintain interest, the lecturer should remember the following key points: conciseness, simplicity, eye contact, variations in speed and volume and the use of personal experience and questions (Mackway-Jones & Walker, 1999).

Skill stations

As CPR involves essentially practical skills, it is important to ensure that any training session allocates plenty of time for these skills to be taught and practised. Skill stations provide an opportunity to learn a skill and debate relevant issues. They should be placed into the context of the overall CPR procedure and be undertaken in small groups (ideally four to six persons). They should take into account, and build on, prior experience and knowledge of the students.

Shared aspects of teaching, learning and prior experience will promote both positive regard and mutual respect. Positive feedback, encouragement and guidance are also particularly important when teaching practical skills.

Mackway Jones and Walker (1999) suggest a four stage approach for teaching a practical skill:

- *The instructor demonstrates the skill at normal speed*: the skill is carried out at normal speed without explanation and commentary, except what would normally be said in the clinical situation. This allows the student to carefully observe the procedure without distraction

- *The instructor demonstrates the skill again, but this time with commentary*: the skill is demonstrated again, but this time with explanation. It will be broken down in small steps, and generally will not be at normal speed
- *The student provides the commentary while the instructor demonstrates the skill*: this stage is used because a skill is more likely to be learned if the student can describe it in detail. If the student is hesitant, the instructor can prompt by leading with the actions. On the other hand confident candidates can describe the different stages of the skill before they are demonstrated. Any errors must be corrected immediately
- *The student demonstrates the skill together with commentary*: each student then talks through and demonstrates the skill. The instructor now has an opportunity to observe each student to ensure they have understood, and are competent at, the skill

Simulated cardiac arrest scenarios

Simulated cardiac arrest scenarios (Figure 17.1) are a further method of teaching CPR skills. They can help to develop team work and help place CPR into context.

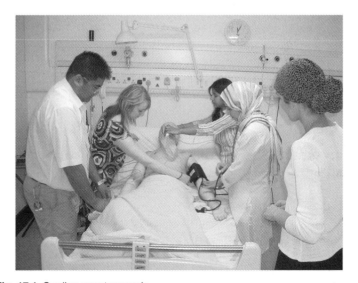

Fig. 17.1 Cardiac arrest scenario.

The scenarios, which should form a major part of any training session, follow on logically from the teaching and practice of individual skills, e.g. bag/valve/mask ventilation, chest compressions and defibrillation. They are a way of putting it all together in a systematic and meaningful way. There are many advantages to this form of training:

- Ideal for training in the clinical area
- Can help to effectively evaluate both an individual and a group performance (Kaye & Mancini, 1986)
- Allow practitioners to practice their skills and to work as a team managing a 'cardiac arrest'
- Can help to bridge the theory/practice gap
- Can increase efficiency and credibility, and improve communication, decision making and team leadership (Basket, 2004)

Discussion groups

Discussion groups, when well organised, are an effective teaching method (Resuscitation Council (UK), 2001). Discussion reflects the method that adults learn best, i.e. it is an active means of acquiring information (Mackway-Jones & Walker, 1999). Active group participation can result in an enjoyable learning experience (Abercrombie, 1989).

It is important to clearly define the desired outcome of the session, e.g. to reach a decision or consensus of opinion (convergent or closed discussion) or to facilitate learners to express and discuss their views (divergent or open discussion) (Resuscitation Council (UK), 2001).

Recommendations for resuscitation training for healthcare staff

The Royal College of Anaesthetists *et al.* (2008) have made the following recommendations for resuscitation training for healthcare staff:

- Staff should undergo regular resuscitation training to a level appropriate for their expected clinical responsibilities

- Staff should be trained use an 'early warning scoring' system to recognise patients at risk of cardiopulmonary arrest and to commence treatment to prevent it (an important component of improving survival in critical illness)
- Training must be in place to ensure that clinical staff can undertake CPR. Training and facilities should ensure that, when cardiopulmonary arrest occurs, staff are able to:
  - ○ Recognise that cardiopulmonary arrest has occurred
  - ○ Summon help (2222)
  - ○ Start CPR using airway adjuncts, and attempt defibrillation within 3 minutes of collapse. This is a minimum standard
- Clinical staff should update their skills annually
- A system must be in place for identifying resuscitation equipment that requires special training, such as defibrillators
- All new members of staff should have resuscitation training as part of their induction programme
- The extension of nursing skills, e.g. to the use of airway adjuncts, intravenous cannulation, rhythm recognition, manual defibrillation and administration of specific drugs in resuscitation, should be encouraged
- Training in resuscitation must be a fundamental requirement for medical and nursing qualifications. Undergraduate and postgraduate examinations for all healthcare workers should include an evaluation of competency in resuscitation
- The resuscitation officer (RO) should organise and coordinate resuscitation training for staff. However, in order to achieve training targets, the RO may need to delegate some aspects of training
- Institutions should recognise and make provision for staff to have enough time to train in resuscitation skills as part of their employment.
- Specific training for cardiopulmonary arrests in special circumstances (e.g. paediatrics, newborn, pregnancy and trauma) should be provided for medical, nursing and other clinical staff in the relevant specialities
- All clinical staff should have the opportunity to attend a multi-professional course in the recognition, monitoring and management of the critically ill patient
- All training should be recorded in a central database

Training mannequins/models

Recent technological advances have enabled the manufacture of life-like training mannequins and models. These are transforming training because a greater number of clinical skills can now be demonstrated and practised in a controlled 'classroom' environment. A general overview of what is currently available will now be detailed.

Airway management models

There is a number of adult airway management mannequins available. Most are anatomically correct in size and detail and benefit from having realistic landmarks including nostrils, tongue, oro- and nasopharynx, larynx, epiglottis, vocal cords, trachea, oesophagus, inflatable lungs and stomach.

Airway management skills that can be demonstrated and practised include the sizing and insertion of the oropharyngeal airway (Guedel airway), suction and tracheal intubation. However it is not possible to realistically perform face mask ventilation on some of the mannequins, as the maintenance of an open airway is not always necessary to achieve chest rise. An adult mannequin is a better alternative.

Resuscitation mannequins

Both basic and advanced full-sized mannequins are now available. Most basic ones can provide detailed and 'real time' feedback. Multifunctional advanced life support mannequins, e.g. SIMMAN (Figure 17.2) are ideal for multi-professional training in the management of an acutely ill patient or a patient in cardiac arrest (Figure 17.3). Common features generally include speech, vital signs, ECG monitoring, basic and advanced airway management including tracheal intubation and emergency cricothyroidotomy, defibrillation, cannulation and drug administration. Practitioners can undertake tasks concurrently providing a more realistic and interactive training session.

Resuscitation Council (UK) courses

The Resuscitation Council (UK)'s Immediate Life Support (ILS) and Advanced Life Support (ALS) Courses are

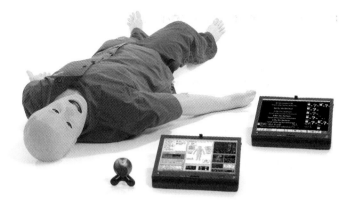

Fig. 17.2 SIMMAN. Reproduced with permission from Laerdal Medical Ltd, Orpington, Kent, UK.

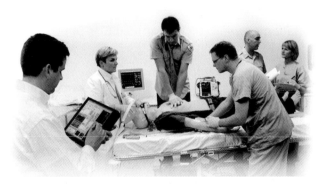

Fig. 17.3 Management of an acutely ill patient or a patient in cardiac arrest. Reproduced with permission from Laerdal Medical Ltd, Orpington, Kent, UK.

nationally and internationally recognised and respected courses.

Resuscitation Council UK Immediate Life Support Course

The Resuscitation Council UK ILS course was developed in order to standardise in-hospital resuscitation training undertaken by ROs; the aim of the course is to train healthcare personnel in CPR, basic airway techniques and safe defibrillation (manual and/or automated external defibrillator (AED)), enabling them to manage patients in cardiac arrest until arrival of a cardiac arrest team and to participate as members of that team (Resuscitation Council (UK), 2009).

Candidates receive the course manual 2 weeks before the course, enabling them undertake pre-course reading/study. The 1-day course comprises of lectures, skills stations, workshops and scenario stations. Assessment of each candidate's performance is undertaken on a continuous basis during the course.

The ILS Course is appropriate for most healthcare professionals who are rarely involved in resuscitation events, but may potentially be the first responders or cardiac arrest team members (Soar *et al.*, 2003); potential candidates include nurses, pre-registration nurses, doctors, medical students, dentists, cardiac technicians, radiographers and physiotherapists (Baskett *et al.*, 2005).

For further information access the Resuscitation Council UK website: www.resus.org.uk.

Resuscitation Council (UK) Advanced Life Support Course

The objectives of the course include teaching the theory and practical skills to effectively manage cardiorespiratory arrest, peri-arrest situations and special circumstances, and preparing senior members of a multi-disciplinary team to treat the patient until transfer to a critical care area is possible (Resuscitation Council (UK), 2009).

An experienced faculty provides a critical illness/cardiac arrest teaching scenario which introduces the concept of role-play and simulated cardiac arrest management, assessment of the critically ill patient, shockable/non-shockable algorithms, positive critiquing and team leadership skills (Resuscitation Council (UK), 2009).

The ALS Course is appropriate for doctors and senior nurses working in emergency care areas and for members of medical emergency and cardiac arrest teams (Nolan, 2001; Royal College of Anaesthetists *et al.*, 2008). For further information access the Resuscitation Council UK website: www.resus.org.uk.

Chapter summary

The importance of resuscitation training has been discussed. CPR skills are generally poor and regular training and re-training are required to ensure that competence and skills are maintained at a satisfactory level. The availability of life-like mannequins and models enables the provision of realistic resuscitation training.

References

Abercrombie M (1989) *The Anatomy of Judgement*. Free Association Books, London.

Basket P (2004) progress of the advanced life support courses in Europe and beyond. *Resuscitation* **62**:311–3.

Baskett P, Nolan J, Handley A *et al.* (2005) European Resuscitation Council Guidelines for Resuscitation 2005: Section 9. Principles of training in resuscitation. *Resuscitation* **67S1**:S181–9.

Broomfield R (1996) A quasi-experimental research to investigate the retention of basic cardiopulmonary resuscitation skills and knowledge by qualified nurses following a course in professional development. *Journal of Advanced Nursing* **23**:1016–23.

Buss P, McCabe M, Evans R *et al.* (1993) A survey of basic resuscitation knowledge among resident paediatricians. *Archives of Disease in Childhood* **68**:75–8.

Fuszard B (1995) *Innovative Teaching Strategies in Nursing*. Aspen, Gaithersburg.

Kaye W, Mancini M (1986) Use of the Mega Code to evaluate team leader performance during advanced cardiac life support. *Critical Care Medicine* **14**:99–104.

Lowenstein S, Libby L, Mountain R *et al.* (1981) Cardiopulmonary resuscitation skills of medical and surgical house officers. *Lancet* **2**:679–81.

Mackway-Jones K, Walker M (1999) *Pocket Guide to Teaching Medical Instructors*. BMJ Books, London.

McKenna S, Glendon A (1985) Occupational first aid training. Decay in CPR skills. *Journal of Occupational Psychology* **58**:109–17.

Moser D, Coleman S (1992) Recommendations for improving cardiopulmonary resuscitation skills retention. *Heart & Lung* **21**:372–80.

Nolan J (2001) Advanced life support training. *Resuscitation* **50**:9–11.

Resuscitation Council (UK) (2001) *Advanced life Support Instructor Manual*. Resuscitation Council (UK), London.

Resuscitation Council (UK) (2009) http://www.resus.org.uk/pages/AtoZindx.htm#c. Accessed 12 July 2008.

Royal College of Anaesthetists, Royal College of Physicians of London, Intensive Care Society & Resuscitation Council (UK) (2008) *Cardiopulmonary resuscitation: standards for clinical practice and training A Joint Statement from The Royal College of Anaesthetists, The Royal College of Physicians of London, The Intensive Care Society, The Resuscitation Council (UK)*. The Royal College of Anaesthetists, London.

Rogers A (1986) *Teaching Adults*. Open University Press, Milton Keynes.

Smith S, Hatchett R (1992) Perceived competence in cardiopulmonary resuscitation, knowledge and skills, amongst 50 qualified nurses. *Intensive and Critical Care Nursing* **8**:76–81.

Soar J, Perkins G, Harris S, Nolan J (2003) The immediate life support course. *Resuscitation* **57**:21–6.

Wynne G, Marteau T, Johnston M *et al.* (1987) Inability of trained nurses to perform basic life support. *British Medical Journal* **294**:1198–9.

Index